8661
11-24-79

D0909092

Health Is Wealth

Books by Paul de Kruif

OUR MEDICINE MEN

MICROBE HUNTERS

HUNGER FIGHTERS

SEVEN IRON MEN

MEN AGAINST DEATH

WHY KEEP THEM ALIVE?

THE FIGHT FOR LIFE

HEALTH IS WEALTH

HEALTH IS WEALTH

BY PAUL DE KRUIF

hb

HARCOURT, BRACE AND COMPANY, NEW YORK

RARE
RA
445
.D39
c.2

COPYRIGHT, 1940, BY
HARCOURT, BRACE AND COMPANY, INC.

COPYRIGHT, 1939, BY
THE CURTIS PUBLISHING COMPANY
IN THE UNITED STATES AND GREAT BRITAIN

*All rights reserved, including
the right to reproduce this book
or portions thereof in any form.*

first edition

Typography by Robert Josephy

PRINTED IN THE UNITED STATES OF AMERICA
BY QUINN & BODEN COMPANY, INC., RAHWAY, N. J.

According to custom —
for Rhea

ACKNOWLEDGMENT

Here is the intimate record of a fight for a national program of human conservation. It began informally as the idea of a small band of Detroit's physicians and public healthmen who are fighting to rid that city of tuberculosis. Its central thought, that health is wealth, was crystallized by Doctor Max M. Peet, who briefly remarked about all those needlessly dying—"it costs much less to save 'em than to bury 'em." Presented persistently during five years in the pages of the *Country Gentleman*, it has aroused nationwide interest. It has failed, so far, in spite of vigorous effort and excellent contacts, to enlist the support of high political leaders. They do not object to the idea. But apparently the public health is not yet for them hot national politics. A large number of men—they include bankers, insurance men, industrialists, a publisher, a lawyer, an advertising executive, public healthmen, physicians, and men of medical science—have made basic contributions to the simple central idea that health is wealth. Thanks to their informal co-working, a national health program has devel-

ACKNOWLEDGMENT

oped. It could be right now written into a non-controversial health law. The names of these co-workers and the parts played by them, are recorded in the book itself. Of their development of the health program the undersigned has been the informal amanuensis. The personal freedom of action to undertake this work is thanks to the generosity and understanding of the officers of the Curtis Publishing Company, and especially to Philip S. Rose.

PAUL DE KRUIF

Pompanocean, Pompano, Florida
February, 1940

CONTENTS

Health Is Wealth

I.   Live or Die

IT IS easy to state the proposition that the health of the people is not controversial. It is simple to say there should be no argument over whether we live or die. It is self-evident that we should all live a life span at a level of vigor that known science can give us. It is not debatable that the span of our lives should grow longer, the level of our energy reach higher as our developing science becomes more powerful. Only cynics, sophomoric, deny this. Only fainthearts believe it impractical. Even these of warped brain and little faith reach out, for themselves and their own, for as much of this life and vigor as their brains and pocketbooks permit. But the mass of us, knowing that for ourselves it is life we hold dearest, do not—deep down—deny life to any other man, woman, or child. We hold this faith to such a degree that we allow our physicians to fight for the sanity and life—even of Al Capone.

Yet today the fight for the health of the people

falls far short of being put into now possible nation-wide action, not action according to the dreams of crackpots, but action based upon plans already prepared by practical, competent men of medical science. Just the same, though the time lag between discoveries and the life-saving use of them is an infamous thing, there are signs that this deadly frustration of science will not be permanent.

From the ranks of physicians and healthmen a new breed of man against death is arising. These men are brothers to humanity and do not despise it. They are coming to guide the mass of the people who want to live. . . .

In the present din of the war of words over the issue of the public health the people do not yet clearly hear the promises of these new men against death, who are modest, and do not yet realize the power of the truth they serve. In the mounting controversy two voices are still dominant, two sides can be seen to be fighting. The one voice is that of medical moss-backs; the other that of the mass of the people—wanting to live. The one is small in numbers. It is made up mainly of men of medicine—some of them highly competent in their profession—who counsel the people to be complacent about the state of their health. These medical leaders point with pride to our

4

low death rate as compared to that of other lands, hinting all is being done that can now be done—

Do they think that the people will rest content to see the highest science used to check the brain syphilis of the derelict Al Capone, while at the same time because of lack of public health science, scores of thousands of innocent babies go on dying from this sinister sickness?

The soothsaying voice of these somewhat old-fashioned doctors is now less and less heard because of the clamor of the second voice, the voice of the people. The insight of the common man and woman looks through and past these reassuring low death rate figures quoted to them by the medical upholders of the public health *status quo*. The fact that slightly fewer babies die a-bornin' than used to die a generation ago—that is no consolation to a father and mother desolate because their own baby has been killed by bad care at life's beginning.

Myriads, diseased and miserable or with their own in danger, now begin to realize the possible boon of discoveries which—if only freely available—could now lift their misery. Or, better still, could have prevented it. The common man and woman know what they want: they want chiefly to live and be strong and vigorous. But the roar of the voice of the millions, demanding this, is yet a confused one. The growing public health pressure groups of the people—formidable at the National Health Conference in 1938 and at the Wagner Health Bill hearings in 1939—were both misled by certain government and labor group visionaries and crackpots. These pseudo-scientists—though well-meaning—seemed to believe the cause of the public health could best be served by snubbing and damning the doctors.

While our doctors—crude though their science may be and limited their skill—are fundamentally the arbiters of life and death of the people.

Now our new men against death are beginning to band to guide the nation's sick and miserable. They are men not of the past or the present but rather of the future. While perhaps not more technically skilled, yet in more than one quality they stand apart from those who are satisfied about present national death rates and today's national vigor. In the light of today's science they do not jubilate over the present state of the health of the nation compared to the awful sickness and death of the old days. If pneumonia, TB, syphilis can be made trivial as causes of death, then they want to begin to make them thus negligible—now. For a people still largely malnourished they refuse to make national vigor appear marvelous by measuring it by yardsticks in use before vitamins were known. If a few wretched ones are today rescued from insanity's doom by new science, then they are irritated that all are not now being saved—all for whom this science holds out hope.

There is another quality of our new men against death most of all fitting them to be leaders in the fight of the people for stronger, fuller, happier life. It is a kind of mercy different from that of the politician complained of by Lincoln. "I suppose the institution of slavery looks small to him," said Father Abraham. "He is so put up by nature, that a lash upon his back would hurt him, but a lash upon anybody else's back does not hurt him." Now it is notable that the slow rot of our present consumptive myriads, the addling of the brains of our hundreds of thousands of daft ones, the torture of the anonymous thousands needlessly dying from cancer—it is significant that all this is pain for our new men against death as well as for the people tormented and suffering.

And the pity of these fighters is practical. They are getting a grasp upon a truth that will soon demand action by politicians upon public health as a national issue. This is the truth that the people's health is the nation's wealth.

I I

The idea of using this plain truth to mobilize new death-fighting power became clear to me in a smoke-dimmed little room over steins of beer in the Detroit Athletic Club in December, 1934. I had been asked to consult with officers of the Detroit Health Department on ways and means to get money to fight tuberculosis. Among the band of men there conspiring was Detroit's health commissioner, Doctor Henry F. Vaughan. He is an engineer, a man absolutely dedicated to downing death rates, something yet new in the fight against death. He is urbane, fighting death rates, not men. For twenty years he has toiled to turn practicing physicians into public healthmen without their losing their identity as private practitioners. Doctor E. J. O'Brien—his hatred of tuberculosis and bitterness against medical incompetence is surpassed only by his skill and fame as a chest surgeon—that evening contributed the fighting spirit to counterbalance Vaughan's suavity. The third important member of that evening's life-plotting triumvirate was

Doctor Bruce H. Douglas. He is a tall thin man, outwardly unemotional, never profane, ginger-ale-drinking and indomitably Quaker. He is Detroit's tuberculosis controller, with immense learning in all phases of the diagnosis and modern treatment of consumption at his finger-tips. These three made a formidable trio.

They had this in common—it is another quality of the new men against death: They were all three convinced the war against TB could not be won, TB could not be stamped out, unless they took full information of their battle to the people. Then how to get the citizens stirred up about the thwarting of science? These three had the weapons in their hands but could not use them. If we could only get Detroit's people sore, indignant about that. . . .

Now Vaughan has a brain-storm. In the midst of our profane table-pounding, beer-drinking— "Michael, some more ginger-ale please for Doctor Douglas!"—Vaughan throws an innocent little problem in public health arithmetic into the discussion which had been getting nowhere fast. Now Vaughan states the problem, then solves it, as follows—

It costs the city of Detroit so many millions of dollars, yearly, to hospitalize its far-advanced tuberculous sick. . . . We will not add in the immense sums needed to bury the victims and give relief to their families. . . . Now it would cost the city a mere fraction of this yearly taxpayers' burden to spot all cases of consumption, early, when still at a stage where a few months, half the present time, in hospital would cure them. This is a task for which Detroit is already superbly equipped. It has progressive physicians, x-ray experts, diagnosticians, chest surgeons, ample hospital beds. So what is lacking?

On the back of a menu card Vaughan—steeped in the figures—sets out the exact millions that TB costs the city. Over against them he writes the exact hundreds of thousands of dollars—which his health department budget has not got—but which would help him find all early cases, cure them, prevent new cases from occurring, rid the city of the white plague.

This is not whimsy or hooey. It is mathematical, scientific, practical. There is only one thing lacking to make—in not much more than a generation's time—this great killer hardly more than an evil memory. What's lacking is a couple of hundred thousand dollars a year to pay the city's doctors, x-ray experts, public health nurses to spot the early cases of consumption. To save the city annual millions of dollars.

Now we forget our beer. We are quiet before the

elegance, the simplicity of Henry Vaughan's demonstration. But can it be made to stir the people? And what popular magazine editor would believe such arithmetic would interest his readers?

Philip S. Rose believed so, and now, in the *Country Gentleman,* early in 1935, the city fathers of Detroit were held up to national scorn for their penny-pinching, their false economy which maintained the tragedy of more than a thousand Detroiters yearly needlessly dying from tuberculosis. For those who are superstitious nothing's more ominous than brilliant success in the opening skirmish of any war. But from the start it seemed as if Vaughan's plan to finance public health on the simple fact that it costs us money to die from preventable disease, must sweep the nation. Hard-bitten Philip S. Rose in his conservative *Country Gentleman* did not hesitate to broadcast the radical news that lost lives are lost money, not only for Detroit, but the nation. Within a year this challenge published in that plain farmer's magazine was accepted by William J. Scripps, of *The Detroit News* and its radio station WWJ.

By November, 1936, amid acclaim of the city's capitalists, doctors, lawyers, preachers and amid enthusiasm of the common people the city fathers took action historic in public health record. To begin to wipe out tuberculosis they passed annual—it was hoped and promised—appropriation of the two hundred thousand dollars Vaughan asked for. To begin to liquidate the burden of yearly millions tuberculosis cost the city's taxpayers.

—It is noteworthy that in this publicity campaign suffering, bereavement, heartbreak were not mentioned. This had the peculiar reverse effect of making the city fathers sentimental—

Those were exciting days. What with President Franklin D. Roosevelt—so solicitous for the welfare of the people—re-elected, what would prevent our spreading Detroit's economic financing of the TB fight to the same method of getting sinews of war for the fight against all preventable sickness and death? Or such was our hope. In the matter of preventable illness it is demonstrable that bad health is bad business. And aren't we a business nation? This idea was presented by our Detroit group to Doctor Thomas Parran, Surgeon General of the United States Public Health Service.

Thomas Parran saw the point of it, so what could stop nationwide adoption of the Detroit plan? At Parran's request, it was presented to over a thousand of the country's healthmen and physicians at the

December, 1936, Conference on Venereal Disease Control Work at Washington, D. C. Wasn't the same silly waste of money apparent in our maintaining millions disabled by gonorrhea and heart-wrecked, underpar, insane from the ghastly luxury of syphilis?

Again the acclaim seemed unanimous. Newspapers, including the conservative *New York Times*, made favorable nationwide editorial comment. Public health, till now a starved orphan among all beneficiaries of today's national spending, now would be cared for, now would be financed, now would be on the march—with what to stop it! In the glow of the day after that conference Doctor Parran made the suggestion that Detroit's economic TB plan be expanded into a national economic health program. How could Congressional budget-balancers dodge it? The President must see the self-liquidating economics, the sense of it.

But we must lay our plans carefully. And so for the better part of the year 1937 the idea that lost lives are lost money was put to a stiff road test. It was kicked around among physicians, industrialists, bankers, healthmen. It was put to an informal poll of public opinion that sampled all levels of the plain people. There was unanimous yes to it, except on the part of one bitterly anti-New Deal Chicago banker. "If preventing disease will save us so many billions at the end of a generation, the Government will find new foolish ways to spend them!" said this die-hard. . . .

But would this make sense to the suffering millions who—for lack of death-fighting money—would sicken and die in the interim?

The *Country Gentleman* now returned to the publicity fight for adequate sinews of war for public health. It published an article, telling the details of how Detroit's people were stirred to demand the needed anti-TB wherewithal. It recommended that the nation apply this common sense to a war against sickness and death. It pointed out that the money Detroit required to abolish the pain and misery of the white plague was, yearly, only 1/400th the cost of one death-dealing battleship.

Toward the end of 1937, it seemed as if the Detroit plan was winning important recognition. The National Tuberculosis Association distributed hundreds of thousands of *Country Gentleman's* story of the fantastic campaign in which Detroit was sold the idea that it was economical to spend death-fighting money. In December, 1937, the time seemed ripe to carry the idea to the President. So now Surgeon

General Thomas Parran and I prepared a two-page memorandum: *Essentials of a National Health Program.*

III

This memorandum assumed that the conservation of the vital resources of the nation is an inherent part of the basic policy of the present Administration.

It stated that, by applying knowledge now available, the immense money losses caused by preventable diseases could be greatly cut down.

It proposed mobilization of a health organization covering every community in the country—but under local control, state supervision, and federal leadership.

It enumerated the now preventable diseases and deaths that could be attacked with scientific weapons of known and unquestioned power to cut down these sickness and death rates.

It asked that the federal government aid the states in the training of the medical profession to fit it to take part in the new program, and to build laboratories, health centers, and hospitals the healthmen and doctors would need in their new great war.

It explained that the medical and allied professions should be made part of the new health army without basic change in our present medical practice.

Not forgetting political angles, the memo ended with assurance that wide public support for the program could be mobilized. Not only from the mass of common citizens, but from the banking, business, and professional interests of the country.

It was an airtight little memorandum that said a mouthful in a few words. But how to get it to the President, not perfunctorily but for his close study? Doctor Parran did not believe it was his role to do this. Of all high government men so far met, Parran has the strictest regard for official punctilio. Not having the lowdown on Washington mysteries, you might think that the Surgeon General of our Public Health Service was a personage of immense power over the nation's life and death. But Parran scoffed at this with a modest smile. "You do not know what a little man I am here in Washington," he said. It did no good to argue that his brilliant fight to bring the menace of syphilis home to the people, that his bold breaking down of the taboo against mention of the sinister sickness, had made him anything but a "little man"—to our citizens.

"But this is not America, it's Washington," said gentle-voiced Parran, with a tolerant smile.

So how to get this preliminary blueprint of a practical health program to our Great White Father? I took the matter up with Mr. Basil O'Connor, former law partner, great and good friend of the President. O'Connor studied the little two-page memo. O'Connor is a notable dead-pan kidder. "What are you excited about?" he asked me. "There is nothing much to this idea. Excepting that it is absolutely sound."

This pat on the back was cause for excitement. O'Connor was one of the nation's ace lawyers. He knew his way round in high financial and political intricacies. He had an immense, disenchanted knowledge of how hard it is to get anything done in a democracy. Here was a powerful recruit for our obscure band of new men against death. Realist and hard-boiled, O'Connor, too, felt the lash of pain of sickness and heartbreak by bereavement that falls on the backs of millions of other people. President of the National Foundation for Infantile Paralysis, he steals more and more of his expensive time for this and other public health hobbies. So, at the beginning of 1938, Basil O'Connor—Doc O'Connor to you—was given the little memo that—so we all hoped—would be great in portent for the health of America.

He said he would do his best. We all waited. For

weeks and months we waited not daring to ask what had happened to our two sheets of paper. And nothing happened. No word. No sign of yes or no or maybe from Washington.

IV

It must be said in justice to the national administration that the President had already begun to show concern for the nation's sick and dying. He had appointed the Interdepartmental Committee to Coordinate Health and Welfare Activities. This comittee's technical medical advisers had submitted an ominous report as a result of its study of the nation's sickness and death to the President at the beginning of 1938. Now the Interdepartmental Committee's Chairman, Miss Josephine Roche, in July, 1938, presided over the famed dog fight known as the National Health Conference, called at Washington by the President, then on cruise in the Pacific.

The conference opened auspiciously and amid the acclaim of the representatives of the people—labor unions, farmers, women's clubs, civic groups—here assembled. . . . Amid the enthusiasm of all but the nation's doctors. . . . "There is nothing more important to a nation than the health of its people," said the President's message read by Miss Roche. This was not debatable. Now public health was coming of age. Now the health of the people was becoming politically hot. "There is need for a co-ordinated national program of action," said the President's message. The conference now proceeded to unco-ordinate itself into bitterly warring factions.

The proposed national health program submitted to the conference by Miss Roche's committee was certainly something. It demanded spending in the grand manner. It proposed far more than our own modest plan of attacking the sickness and death rates of disease now preventable, curable. It suggested a gigantic plan of medical care for the famous one third of a nation. It outlined a federal doctoring scheme for the many additional millions to whom sickness may without question at any time become financial disaster. The lay groups present at the conference were in general uncritically enthusiastic. The program made front page headlines all over the country. The sums proposed to finance this medical care plan were astronomical—and no technique for raising this money nor for liquidating the expenditure was presented.

Now the fat was in the fire. Distinguished representatives of the American Medical Association rose to make indignant protest. Their protest—alas—put the nation's doctors on a nasty spot. With all lay groups unanimous for a national health program, why, just why, should the doctors be against this particular one? It was easy to insinuate that the A.M.A. was against all health programs. It was so insinuated. In justice to the physicians it must be here stressed that they had not been consulted by Miss Roche or her medical brain trust. There were compulsory health insurance advocates on her committee who held the A.M.A. in contempt. . . .

Now the effort to arrive at preliminary agreement on ways and means to expand the nation's health activity turned into a shindy. There was something weird, something screwball about this schoolboyish wrangling over matters as grave as life and death. . . . And something unnecessary, on both sides unnecessary. Doctor Olin West, General Manager of the American Medical Association, advised those here assembled "to put a brake on their thinking and not try to make the world over in a day."

The Association's President, Doctor Irvin Abell, protested that this vast scheme for centrally controlled medical service could not possibly be approved of by public health administrations.

Against the indignant doctors an utterly non-medical force opposed itself. Lawyer Lee Pressman of the C.I.O.—there is small doubt the C.I.O. was powerful in the Interdepartmental Committee— made a grave accusation. "When I criticize the medical associations," Pressman cried, "I do not criticize individual physicians, but the upper hierarchy who refuse to heed the needs of the poor or their own colleagues who lack patients."

This was equivalent to accusing the A.M.A. brass hats of being accessories before the fact of the needless dying of American citizens.

Probably Lawyer Pressman did not realize that when he attacked their officials, he was in effect attacking the country's doctors. Among all our country's organizations of workers—dungaree or white collar—there is no other with a guild spirit, a solidarity so deep, so ancient as that of the doctors. Now putting the finger on their leaders, Pressman was, though not meaning to, denouncing one hundred and thirteen thousand doctors as stony-hearted in the matter of life or death.

Doctor Morris Fishbein—as *quick* a thinker on his feet as there is in America—made a shrewd thrust at the Roche health proposals when he pointed out that health was not the country's primary problem. "Let us concern ourselves first with that question of food,

fuel, clothing, shelter, and a job at adequate wages,"
urged this most famous of medical orators. You could
get his meaning. A large part of the people have
today not got these fundamentals. Why should a
government, unable to supply them after five years
of trying, planning, now begin to monkey with large
scale plans for public health?—which was good in
our country—compared to that of other peoples! Of
course there are those in the front line trenches of the
war against death and misery who are qualified to
protest that Doctor Fishbein—in the passion of controversy—was a bit lyrical over our public health
status quo. Impartial inquiry would reveal a legion
of millions of miserable ones—but millions—who if
they had heard him would mutter that the good doctor was drawing a long bow when he told the conference—

"You are an essentially healthful people."

What was the net result of this comedy of contention over the tragedy of America's sick and suffering?
Who had drawn up the grandiose Roche health
plan? Anybody but the doctors of the country. Did
the country need and was it beginning to demand expanded public health and medical care activity?
Without question, yes. But who must care for the
nation's sick? Its doctors and nurses. Who can begin

the now possible cutting down of the sickness and death rates? Only our medical scientists, doctors, and nurses—all co-working with our public healthmen.

Why was it that, at the time of the conference, neither Surgeon General Parran nor representatives of the American Medical Association were planners on the Interdepartmental Committee?

The net result of the conference was that the American people had less faith in the army that alone could fight for its higher level of health.

V

Now 1938 drew toward its close with action on a national health program farther away than ever. It was bitter for our obscure, anonymous, unorganized band of new men against death. The more so because we knew that the enthusiasm of the people for this one good war against mankind's ultimate enemy was obvious, was growing. Even Congress had shown itself ready for action. This very Spring the Venereal Disease Control Bill had passed both houses of Congress without a dissenting vote. Yet this isolated legislation—even for syphilis and gonorrhea it was inadequate—was trivial in the face of what the nation's sick and miserable needed, in the face of what a sound, workable health program could do for them. Yet this action by Congress, and also its passage of the Cancer Control Act—even though that too was a drop in the bucket—showed that public health could cut clean across party lines. So now—

If the economic public health program could only be got to the top, to the President. If it only could be made—political. But political in the highest meaning.

—What folly, with all of us distrustful of politics and none of us politicians!—

And yet, and but, in a democracy no measure becomes law unless it is first political. Naively the drive now began to make the life or death of the people a matter, not of politics, but statesmanship. In the elections of 1938 the administration had suffered severe reverses. In Washington there were wisecracks about the need of a new rabbit to be produced from the New Deal's battered hat. But wasn't our health plan exactly that rodent? It seemed double-barreled in its power and political appeal. It would save the lives of voters. They had no objection. It would save do-re-mi for the taxpayers. They had long been groaning about national waste of money.

"Boy, you've got something there. It looks to me like a natural." So said Works Progress Administration's Howard O. Hunter. Now Hunter, able administrator, hard-boiled politician, was a skilled and dogged fighter for and devotee of the public health. Now through his interest a conference was arranged for Doctor Parran and me, with Harry L. Hopkins, head of W.P.A. and famed as the friend of America's underdog millions. Hopkins could not help being sympathetic to a sound plan for action to lift the nation's sickness and misery. He was—more important still—one of the President's close friends and advisers.

Hopkins showed his sympathy and interest by giving us a whole morning of his valuable time. Thomas Parran—as always insisting what a little man he was in Washington and not realizing himself what a big man he was becoming in the country— now helped, with his diffidence, his usual terrific modesty, to give the genial Hopkins the lowdown on what right now was possible. Hopkins, amiable, slouchy, informal in an old red dressing gown but with a direct wire to the White House at his elbow, was patient and honest with us. Without saying so he managed to convey to us that the hour of the fight against death had not yet struck. This did not daunt us from trying to sell our magic rabbit.

He was enlightened about how evil it was that the

American Medical Association had become a so-and-so with the Government, and vice versa. He was told how the physicians of the country need not be antagonized, but could on the contrary be enlisted for a health war that was sound, economic, good for their prestige and pocketbooks as well as for the lives and the balance sheet of the nation. At the drop of a hat, at a word from the President, it would be possible to assemble at Washington a little committee, commission—whatever you wanted to call it—of distinguished men of medicine and public health. They were not politicians of either party or the medical variety. They would not wrangle. They would not recriminate. They would sketch for the President the possibilities, they would define the practical limitations of the new war against death. They would be men not only highly competent, each one, in his own medical discipline, but *persona grata* to organized medicine. Not one would have an ax to grind. All would be bound by faith that the public health is far greater than any man working for it—

Harry Hopkins listened. His interest encouraged us.

The committee need not consist of much more than a dozen individuals, all of top rank, each a practical fighter of disease and death in his own field. There would be no theorists, crackpots, chasers of public health rainbows in this bunch. They would be bold tough men in contrast to Washington's too abundant supply of hesitant, liberal, yes-but men—

Men of the stamp of Paul O'Leary of the Mayo Clinic, against syphilis, and Walter M. Simpson of Dayton, Ohio, against gonorrhea.

E. J. O'Brien of Detroit, co-planner of the economic health program, famed chest surgeon and implacable and practical, against tuberculosis.

Even James Ewing—grand old man against cancer—could be pressed into service despite his age.

J. G. M. Bullowa of New York was not only hard-boiled in his testing of remedies against pneumonia, but for him the disease was a public health challenge.

Dynamic Elliott C. Cutler, of Harvard, had a new slant on surgery—since formidable national death from bad surgery gives that discipline a public health angle.

Who would be abler in recommending expansion of medical research and education, demanded by a sound health program, than George Whipple, Nobel Prize-man from Rochester, New York?

The fight for the lives of mothers and new-born babies could find no wiser and more practical planner than Beatrice E. Tucker, Director of De Lee's famed Maternity Center in Chicago.

William F. Lorenz, of Madison, Wisconsin, looked at insanity as disease, physical disease even though ordinarily called mental. He had sound views of how to make beginning of emptying our asylums.

Diseases caused by sub-visible viruses were looming more and more important in the health fight and Thomas M. Rivers of the Rockefeller Institute could advise on not only scientific but practical plans in this sector.

The marvelous life-saving possibilities of the new magic coal-tar chemicals—like sulfanilamide—were best known, not only from the scientific but plain doctors' angle, by Perrin H. Long of the Johns Hopkins Medical School.

If the task of public health organization involved in the new health program should be formidable for Surgeon General Parran—who would be a more sagacious and bolder counselor than Karl F. Meyer of San Francisco?

There would be need for cordial understanding between organized medicine and the national administration. Max M. Peet of Ann Arbor, Michigan—devoted to the President and famed and respected by physicians from coast to coast—could serve in this key position.

The food of the people is now fundamental in every sector of the death fight. William De Kleine of the American Red Cross was fit for this task of making nutrition basic in public health.

Mind you, the men here named were singled out from a much larger panel of the new kind of men against death. It must be explained that this committee was proposed to Mr. Hopkins by myself, not by Doctor Parran, though the personnel of it in general had his respect and confidence. They would be powerful because they were a unit in devotion to a common aim. They were all occupied in such important posts that none could be suspected of ambition to become a jobholder in the government. Theirs was a patriotism—for the public health and for America—to permit the sacrifice of a part of their time from research, and teaching, and their practices to become members of an informal general staff for the new war against death. They could be thought of as a Praetorian Guard for Surgeon General Parran, whom it was hoped the President would choose to lead the national health program.

The selection of such a group of practical men by the President would do much to close the present breach between the government and organized medicine. It was absurd to pretend that the country's doctors were less anxious than any other group of citizens to prevent sickness and death. Surely Mr. Hopkins realized that it was only by using our practitioners of medicine as front line soldiers—giving them a chance for training but not disturbing their ancient rights—that a workable health program could be put into effect.

Mr. Hopkins was given the works that morning. No trick was missed, no bet overlooked, no argument forgotten. It would not be hard to organize pressure groups to show Congress that this was a fight in which everybody wins. The people were at this moment in advance of their leaders in their demand—or their readiness to demand—the right to live.

That morning we went all out. And at the end of it Mr. Hopkins asked for a memorandum. He was not encouraging. He was honest and hinted no promises. His information about plans for the 1939 budget indicated that it would hardly permit financing of a health program—even the modest one here put forward. That deflated us. But there was yet one card to be played. There was an ace in the hole. Would Mr. Hopkins object if Mr. Marriner S. Eccles, Chairman of the Federal Reserve Board, should pass upon the soundness—long range economic—of the proposed health plan? There might be ways—even permissible by the nation's money power which is not at Washington!—by which the needed funds could be obtained outside the budget. . . .

Mr. Hopkins said it would be fine to get the reaction of Mr. Eccles to an economic health program. That morning Mr. Hopkins was an excellent listener. Yet his kindly parting pat on the back conveyed the feeling to me that, amid the terrific issues of unemployment, the persisting economic tailspin, the threat of world war, our proposed fight for the nation's health and lives was—minor league stuff, strictly speaking.

That evening Marriner Eccles studied the memorandum—slightly more detailed than the one approved ten months before by Basil O'Connor. It was a lift to hear Eccles say that it was economically sound. It was stirring to hear Eccles suggest that he knew a possible way to raise the money—extrabudgetary—to start this good war that in the long pull would not only save lives but vast sums of money. This was one of those high evenings reminiscent of the stirring days of November, 1936, when Detroit's city fathers approved Henry Vaughan's TB-fighting budget.

What now could stop the health program? The Chairman of the Federal Reserve Board approved it, and was willing to help with the all-important financing of it. The President's close friend and adviser, Hopkins, was friendly to it. And the President—?

The next evening of this mid-November, 1938, we prepared a super-condensed memorandum—for transmission by Mr. Hopkins. It was titled MEMORANDUM TO THE PRESIDENT. It was one page long—double-spaced. It told him that the most neglected phase of his program was the conservation of the country's human resources, and that this conservation was essential to the national defense, would aid employment, and would contribute to the general economic welfare of the nation. It suggested that such a program of human conservation could be quickly placed on a level with that of national defense and of soil conservation, and that it would receive more nearly unanimous support than any of the other great objectives the President had sponsored in our national life. It suggested that the President call a small group together—including Henry Morgenthau and Marriner Eccles—for detailed discussion of the implications of this memorandum.

"Just as the country first turned toward you in

your championship of the forgotten man, it will turn toward you again if you champion this forgotten issue."

It was on this note the memorandum ended. The following morning it was dispatched to Mr. Hopkins. Nothing has ever been heard of its reception or its ultimate fate.

VI

What was there left to do but go back to the typewriter, what else after this futile foray on the fringes of high politics? What to do but go back to Wake Robin, to the sun house high over the sand that sings under your bare feet in summer, that cuts your face when it's whipped by the northwest gales of November that blow up echelons of steel-gray white-capped combers, pounding on the beach, shaking the sun house? What to do but sit poking through the last three years of data about life and death, the notes, the hopeful stories of Detroit's TB death fight, which we thought it was going to be duck soup to spread to the health of the nation.

—Now came ominous news. Richard Reading, the budget balancing Mayor of Detroit, in the name of economy, was out to slash the TB appropriation that

33

was going to result in the city's most notable economy—

So what now to do but wool-gather through the
eleven windows of the sun house shaking under the
northwest gales and the white and steel-gray surf,
spending mornings staring at the straight line made
by the dark water and the gray-clouded sky. It is a
simple line, impersonal and timeless. It makes all
fret and worry over questions of living and dying
seem—dated. Winter, Spring, Summer, and now
again into this present fag end of November, Lake
Michigan goes through her cycle that began before
there were men and that will continue after mankind
has gone. Why worry? If the people want life, they
will live. The breaking up of the ice in April when
the high air is full of the warble of north-flying blue-
birds brings hopes again. Maybe in the Spring we'll
wangle a way to the man in the White House. . . .

Hopes are highest, energy is tops when the sun is
strong and the water green blue and gentle in July,
but here it is only November with the bleak gray
omen of the lake that will soon be dead silent, dead
white with the ice of Winter, the death of Winter.
Yet, even now, the human battery recharges under
Lake Michigan's majesty, impersonality, and in a
couple of weeks it sends you back into the battle.

Doctor O. C. Wenger—field commander of the fight by the United States Public Health Service against syphilis—makes anybody ashamed to say die in this war for the health of America. Philip Rose never gives up, keeps saying no national issue he has fought for in the *Country Gentleman* has ever failed of adoption, finally. With these two, Rhea and I now had a conference in Chicago at the end of November, 1938. Some might think it futile to return to the fight through the pages of this farmers' paper, to go back to hammering for a health program on those slick white pages instead of on the rough paper of the highbrow weeklies or monthly periodicals that reach "the people who think," the "intelligent people who count for something in this country." But at this Chicago conference O. C. Wenger thinks it's great, fine, wonderful—the more millions know of life now possible, the better; and the plainer and stronger those millions who spell out the simple statement of a now possible, practical health program, the more powerful will be the pressure— finally—surging up to Washington from the bottom.

Why, we haven't even made the plain statement of a health program so far. So let's go. Let's write something to put the responsibility up to the politicians.

At this conference Phil Rose listened with narrowed eyes to our scheme for an open letter to the President, to be published in the *Country Gentleman*. The people are far in advance of their leaders in wanting strength and life—even though they're still not articulate in demanding it. Congress would not block it. The government could make peace with the doctors and gain their absolutely indispensable co-operation. The President has gone on record saying, last July: "There is nothing more important to a nation than the health of its people." So why not smoke out the President?

Rose listens with dead pan, narrow-eyed. Look, not only the people, the public healthmen, the doctors are ready to go. The bankers can be brought along to get back of the necessary expenditures that will result in such vast national economy. Public financiers like Eccles, brilliant private bankers like First Boston Corporation's George D. Woods have passed on the soundness of the economic health program. Here's the line to take in this open letter: Human life is the greatest of all American resources, Mr. President. These resources are now in a state of erosion. Death does not wait, Mr. President, and this being a democracy, you are our servant, we are not your slaves, and we have a right to tell you. It is wasteful to wait. It is heartless to dally—

O. C. Wenger, loving trouble, irritating imp of public health that he is, believes that this is a swell idea. He will aid in making any mischief to get the cause of the public health more talked about, so that the scandal of needless dying will be better broadcast. Questions of discretion, of taste, are nothing to Wenger who with wrecked heart lives in that good company of men who know their days are numbered, who go to bed never sure they will wake up next morning. He is now all for cooking up a strong stew and placing the dish on the doorstep of 1600 Pennsylvania Avenue, Washington, D. C.

At last Phil Rose speaks. He says no. Our hearts are heavy that moment. No, he will not publish an open letter to the President in the *Country Gentleman*. No, it is not for us to tell the President. But it is for us to tell the people, the two millions who subscribe, the many millions who read this farm paper. And we haven't been telling him one story, but two. The first is the story of America's needless human erosion. It will smoke out those who congratulate us on what a healthy people we are, who say hurrah for the *status quo*, whose words are a narcotic of complacency. The second story can tell today's possibility of human conservation, how disease can now be prevented, eliminated, and how, if that is done, the total energy of the people will be enormously increased.

"So go on and write those stories. But not to the President," said Phil Rose. "Tell them to the American people."

Wenger was jubilant. Here, instead of one story going out to the millions, was the chance for two. So ended discouragement over the fiasco of political finagling for public health. So now I could go back to my proper work at the typewriter, to the job of agitating the people. "It is clear that from the blue waters of Lake Michigan and its white sandy shore you have gathered strength and perspective for the long pull which will be needed for the job ahead of us," wrote Thomas Parran. It was stirring that he felt there was a job ahead for all of us. "It is true that for a health program, we should have the whole country as a pressure group," wrote Parran. "Unfortunately, however, people do not yet realize the specific impact of public health measures on them as individuals. It is always the other fellow who is apt to be sick, to get tuberculosis or to contract pneumonia."

There was the job. How to do my own bit to begin to build the pressure group of 130,000,000 for the one fight in which everybody wins? How to burn the beauty and the glory, the need for this one good war, into you and you and you?

So Phil Rose and Wenger, Thomas Parran and Rhea dictated the job to be done, made it possible to forget the folly of my ride on the Washington merry-go-round. It is not the politicians, it is the people who will—in the long pull—say whether they'll live or die. So two stories, *Human Erosion* and *Human Conservation*, were prepared for publication in the *Country Gentleman*. In an expanded form they are here presented.

II. Human Erosion *

IT HAS taken a long time for this question of live or die to become a political issue. In 1776 the Continental Congress in immortal words—but words—held it to be self-evident that all men are endowed with certain unalienable rights, that among these are Life, Liberty, and the pursuit of Happiness. Now, at the beginning of 1939, our Congress is about to be asked to face today's erosion of our human resources, to consider legislation that will begin nationwide human conservation. Can practical means be found to help our physicians and healthmen give the people the strength and the length of life science without question now can give them?

Congress is going to be asked to face what ought to be self-evident truth: that human conservation is as fundamental as saving of the land, the woods, and other natural resources. Human conservation is no less basic than our obligation to defend our land against foreign invaders.

* Substantially as printed in *Country Gentleman*, March 1939.

To those who object that there are now more serious political questions this must be admitted: that a truly healthy nation must remain a dream so long as millions are jobless, so long as the present mysterious dead hand remains on the productive power of the people. But aren't we maybe putting the cart before the horse? Shouldn't we begin to apply the one science we *know* has power to the people's productive potential? Economists from Adam Smith to Karl Marx have turned out to be false prophets. The word "science" applied to economics is laughable. But if medical science were permitted to be turned on full strength to make the mass of the people strong, even if a Pasteur of economics has not yet come, wouldn't the people in their new vigor demand him?

Winter, 1938, at Harris Neck in McIntosh County, Georgia, malaria-fighter M. E. Winchester gave Rhea and me a primitive example of the economic power of public health. He quizzed Negro farmer Henry Sallens. How did it feel to be rid of malaria? (This had thinned his blood, sapped his strength—lifelong—till in 1937 atabrine had cured him, then prevented re-infection.) Sallens answered, very slow: "Now I feel like working. For the first time I *want* to work." He drew himself up to his height of six feet. "This farm ain't enough to keep me busy. There's an oyster factory down by the river. Been closed couple of years. Bad management, they say. We all want to work there. Why does there have to be bad management? We want to work. Make some real money."

The fires of his energy, only smoldering for forty years, were beginning to glow. And if medical science started now to make our millions of Sallenses—black and white—really strong, if it began to bring them to life's full vigor, would they go on taking the politicians' and the bankers' alibis about there not being enough work for everybody? Or would they arise to demand the right to work that is as basic as the right to live? The people will be slow to unite to demand the unleashing of full productive power —so long as myriads are needlessly sick, needlessly deteriorated, with scores of millions hardly more than half-alive.

Now at the beginning of 1939, our Congress is to be asked to consider legislation for an adequate national health program, and already there are rumblings about coming arguments, of a lobby led by Publisher Frank Gannett—to rally the doctors against the passing of a national health law. It is going to be socialistic. It is going to mean regimentation of the nation's doctors. It will bring into being that horrible bogey—state medicine. So the coming discussion of ways and means toward human conservation is going to raise fierce arguments.

About facts there can be no argument. If two facts are faced, never for a moment lost sight of, then nationally we can unite for action. The first is that human erosion in our country is appalling and widespread. The second is that rebuilding of a great part of this deteriorated humanity is in our power—with no basic change in relation of patients and doctors, with no damage to our democratic way of life.

II

If you get around over our country, if you put your ear to the ground, it becomes clear that the people are becoming restless about the more and more glaring fact of their own erosion. When they are told, "You are an essentially healthy people," they may not yet express mass resentment at such soothsaying, but a sharp ear can already detect a sinister murmur of the people's bitter laughter. Of course they know that their doctors and healthmen have won partial victories over certain sicknesses. In the past generation there has been a downing of death rates—of TB, diphtheria, typhoid fever, some diseases of children. Yet there is hardly a family in the land which isn't now, or which hasn't been, or which tomorrow may not be blighted by sickness—preventable or curable. And a great proportion of such families—if you're interested and have the nerve to listen through to the end—have gruesome stories to tell. Of invalidism, of life-wreck, of death due to their failure—for one reason or another—to get the medical, the public health care that science now knows how to give them.

—It does not solve the problem to lament about the mass of the people being too stupid to take advantage of the wonderful facilities now at their disposal—

And it is fair to ask if it is not Publisher Gannett and his cohort of defenders of the nation's health *status quo* who are the stupid ones? Or worse—when they point with pride at the front of our house of health, ignoring the termites of human deterioration and disease that gnaw within it. Beneath the surface of our nation's alleged essential health, there is a dry rot of damaged human protoplasm. There is human suffering, pain, misery, physical degeneration, needless dying, and half-life worse than death. And one of these days a John Steinbeck is going to arise to depict its horror, its scandal. Ballyhoo about our low general death rate as compared to that of other peoples, pictures of progress of public health against certain sicknesses—these do not alter the totality of our people today sick and deteriorated—with more than half of our nation less than half-alive.

Seventy thousand of our people still die yearly from tuberculosis. But out of 130 millions that is maybe not so many. You point to the decline during the past generation in TB's death rate. Marvelous. And yet, as a murderer of Americans between ages 15 and 45, the tuberculosis microbe is surpassed only by accidents. You say tuberculosis has dropped to seventh place in the big league of America's killers. Congratulations. Yet for every one of the seventy thousand yearly dying, five others are sick with consumption. This totals 420,000 coughing, hemorrhaging, feeble, rotten-lunged, bed-ridden burdens on our commonwealth. You may add to these some unknown hundreds of thousands whose consumption has been "arrested"—but who cannot do a man's or a woman's proper work, who must live half-lives, and are not vigorous citizens.

Such is our essential health in respect of tuberculosis.

Scoffing that this is not yet a formidable percentage of our 130 million, you may be asked to remember another lung-sick cohort. Pneumonia kills more than one hundred thousand people yearly. And since only one out of three, threatened with its strangling agony, dies of it, a total of three hundred thousand of our people are unable to work for weeks or months, or are wrecked for a longer time by resulting pleurisy, or are put out of action for good and all.

So we approach our first million of citizens who cannot be called essentially healthy. Now to these we can add those cancerous. Cancer is not scoffed at even by the most complacent. Terror of it is justified by reason of the one hundred and forty thousand it yearly kills, and this annual death toll is growing. Now for every one of these yearly dying from cancer, several others are sick, in pain, or bed-ridden from its torture, or knocked out by operations that are designed to cure them or wrecked by the suffering often resulting from the x-ray and radium that may be the only hope for them, or gnawed by worry about these cures that still have such a good chance of failing.

Now we approach the second million of American citizens not essentially healthy. Now another and particularly pitiful annual class of recruits for our country's unhealthy rearguard must not be forgotten. These are the gibbering, vacant-eyed battalions of the mentally sick—at this moment more than 500,000 of them crowd our asylums. You may argue that we are now more finicky about calling people normal, that we're quicker than we used to be about judging them legally crazy. Maybe. But this is counterbalanced by the situation in states where only the absolutely mentally helpless or homicidally dangerous are admitted to asylums—because beds do not exist for the treatment of those in the earlier or milder phases of mental sickness. The menace is growing. The number of people in hospitals for the mentally sick went up by forty per cent between 1926 and 1936. You say there are none such in your family? Yet it is estimated by such an authority as Doctor Morris Fishbein that out of 2,144,800 babies born in 1936, eventually 110,000 to 120,000 will be committed to hospitals for mental disease.

In short—one out of twenty of that year's human cohort will be brain-sick enough to have to spend time in a mental institution.

Then besides—according to Doctor Henry A. Luce—there are several times this legally insane 500,000 who are at large, definitely psychotic and many of them dangerous or unreliable or suffering from psycho-neuroses. There are millions of such people—number not precisely estimated—who cannot be said to be reliable, vigorous, productive citizens; who cannot be counted as possible defenders of the nation in wartime.

All these subtract further millions from our essentially healthy America.

The blood test dragnets now being swept through so many communities by healthmen and doctors make it clear that more than 5,000,000 of our people carry the blood taint of syphilis. Indeed, recent figures indicate that this number is nearly one out of twenty of our population—close to 6,500,000. Of course a great part of these infected people are not obviously sick. It is true that syphilis often gnaws silently, far under a seeming healthy exterior. It is true again that syphilis kills only some 50,000 people yearly, with heart-wreck, and that its last horrible consequence, insanity, accounts for only about ten per cent of all first admissions to our asylums. Granted. Again it must be admitted that there are only roughly 60,000 babies born alive—though ghastly caricatures of new humanity—with syphilis, yearly. And there are not more than a few score thousands of youngsters who, because of syphilis, go toward man- and womanhood with dimming eyes.

And yet of the totality of syphilitic six-odd millions, how many are underpar because of this blood taint? How many are lacking in energy, feeble in thought, unfit for work because—gnawed by the secret of their condition—they worry over its sinister promise?

In short, in our alleged healthy America, would you go to that six-odd million of syphilitic Americans for soldiers or sailors, or for transport pilots, or truck drivers, or precision workers in industry that's the foundation of our more and more highly mechanized society?

Would you choose among this tainted cohort for your husband or wife? Of this six million, how many —because of the rigors of the now available treatment—stick with that treatment long enough to be returned to the ranks of America's healthy?

Even at life's beginning, when life should be lusty and strong, the condition of American mothers, bearers of that life, cannot be viewed with too much gratification. It is true that here there have been some public health advances, and that only some twelve thousand American women yearly die from the immediate consequences of childbirth. Yet it is estimated that some 200,000, in addition, become invalids as their reward for bringing life to our nation. And just as life is not kind to hundreds of thousands of mothers, so it is denied to 75,000 babies stillborn yearly. And it is cut short for another 70,000 carried out in little white coffins within the first few weeks of their arrival on earth.

This catalog of doom may be seemingly lightened by one item of which our doctors and healthmen are proud—namely, the progress in conquest of the diseases and death of childhood. Here the forces of human conservation have begun to concentrate formidable power. Even so, every year, among the supposedly healthy millions of our young America— aged one month to fifteen years—140,000 die. For each one dying, many are stricken but survive the maladies of childhood. Many recover without trace of permanent injury. Yet, for others, death would have been preferable. Many recover, and live, but that's all. Hundreds of thousands, damaged by rheumatic fever and other infections, remain marred for life, in their hearts, kidneys, nervous systems. They are left at the post in the stern race to earn their livings.

To the millions already counted, other cohorts must be added—with strength sapped by malaria, twisted and pain-racked by the rheumatism of gonorrhea, with silicosis, pellagra, and with hearts and nervous systems wrecked by a hidden hunger for vitamins lacking in the food of undernourished, mal-nourished millions. Many of these do not even show up in the morbidity rates. Yet they cannot be counted among the truly living. They all add to the rollcall of our national infamy. Their human condition is infamous because their suffering is, by now known science, either eradicable or to a greater or less degree controllable.

Nothing has been said, up till now, of that twisted, crippled army of arthritics—whose mass disability in the wage-earning period of their lives is greater than that caused by any other sickness. Then, to complete the panorama of our allegedly vigorous population, millions of people in middle life, or just past it, must not be forgotten. The hearts, the blood vessels, the brains of these are hit by high blood pressure or hardening of the arteries. The recent National Health Survey estimates the number of these at some 3,700,000.

Hay fever is a joke—to those not afflicted by it—and asthma may be dismissed as a minor cause of death—yet more than 3,000,000 of our people breathe with difficulty because of these afflictions, and during their illness cannot be said to be essentially healthy.

Of course there is a certain degree of overlapping

in this grim catalog of an unfit America. Many, tuberculous, are also arthritic, and so forth. Even so there have been here enumerated a sufficient number of millions to give the other side of the rosy picture of a healthy America. This is what you find when you go beyond the beautiful low death rate reports on one single sickness. These are the myriads of a totality of deterioration that makes you stop your ears if you listen long enough to this rollcall of suffering and misery. Here is a grim army of half-humanity which, if it had the strength to parade before us, would stretch from coast to coast. This is the human erosion that strikes—in one form or another—into every home in America.

This is the new frontier to be opened by the pioneering energy of our new men against death. If they could be taken into the councils of our politicians, if they could have authoritative voice in those councils, if our leaders—political and industrial—united to rebuild America with the simple and single object of raising America's level of vigor—there would be full time work for all for as many years as all today will live. . . .

III

Political leaders being what they are, it is certainly too much to hope that their policies will soon be determined by the science of biology, of medicine, and of public health. Yet today the deeds of our men against death—thwarted though they are—have already begun to light the imagination of the people. Hasn't the time come for these soundest of all leaders, with the help of the people, to get a foot in the door of the councils of our statesmen? If the facts of today's deterioration, of physical degeneration, are nightmares, we can already do more than shudder with fear of them. There are opposing facts, equally true, and more hopeful than any in our nation's history. There exists today a great potential body of volunteers for a new army of human conservation.

These are our biologists, founding the new science of human ecology—the study of the relation of man to his environment. These are our searchers, men of mercy, healthmen and doctors, not yet organized but ready to serve in a mass attack on sickness and death rates in a nationwide fight for life. In a thousand laboratories, in far-flung health departments, in homes, in hospitals from coast to coast they fight brilliant, though handicapped, isolated battles against many forms of human erosion.

And they are in the best sense, and in all meanings of the term, human economists. They have Yankee ingenuity. Where formerly they might save tens with expensive science, now they begin to save hundreds of thousands with weapons keener, more practical, cheaper. By the x-ray's magic eye they can now pick up the first faint threat of tuberculosis. At first this x-ray was far too costly to be applied to the mass-finding of consumption. Now comes news of an x-ray lens that will cut down the cost of looking for TB's danger to 10 cents per person.

The cost of fighting syphilis with arsenical and bismuth drugs in a long-drawn-out, dangerous, and painful treatment has been formidable. The average time needed for cure has been eighteen months. Now comes the massive-dose drip treatment to cure early stages of syphilis in five days. And if this treatment is yet too dangerous for general use, artificial fever— now safe and controllable—when combined with small doses of arsenical drugs can be used for a rapid, powerful and vastly less expensive cure of syphilis.

Not more than three years ago there was no certainly effective treatment for gonorrhea, a vastly disabling and widespread disease, wrecking the lives of hundreds of thousands of women, twisting the limbs of other thousands in the most exquisite of all rheumatic torture. Now—if a medical-health army were mobilized against it—by means of sulfanilamide or artificial fever or a combination of both—this plague could be brought under control.

Pneumonia, a few years ago fatal to one out of three of all stricken with it, now in a high proportion of cases succumbs to serums so powerful that many apparently doomed people are cured in a few hours. But serum is very expensive. Human life is maybe too cheap to permit the cost of a hundred dollars to save it. Now comes sulfapyridine, the relatively cheap magic chemical, the expert use of which could make pneumonia sink to negligible rank from its present position of the nation's third killer—at a cost of six dollars *per capita*.

Cancer, caught early and in parts of the body accessible to the surgeon's knife, or skillfully treated by x-ray or radium, now loses its terror at least to the extent that people begin to speak without voices hushed with dread—about cancer. Though it must be granted that safe and powerful cancer treatment is still highly expensive.

The science and art of obstetrics are now so highly developed that among 18,000 deliveries of women in the filthy slums of Chicago, the death rate of mothers is six times lower than the maternal mortality of the nation as a whole. The improvement in their technique of obstetrical science by Chicago's doctors—thanks to the death fight led by Health Commissioner Herman Bundesen—has cut the rate of dying of newborn babies far below that of the average for the nation, and below that of any large city in the world.

The imbecilic doom that awaits all but a few of the hundreds of thousands contracting the mental disease, dementia praecox—now crowding our asylums with eighty per cent of their incurables—can be fought, with cure or improvement for many, by the new insulin and metrazol shock treatments. The melancholia of women at change of life can now often be nipped in the bud by skillful use of the new sex hormones. The pellagrous insane—and certain malnourished crazy people without sign of pellagra—can be brought back to clearheadedness in a few days by the chemical magic of the cheap vitamin, nicotinic acid.

Such is a part of the power of new medical science. It is already in action. But only against an infinitesimal fraction of our human erosion. Each of these discoveries is a true story of hope for myriads of stricken ones. Each today remains a story with an unhappy ending. Because this new life must be denied to millions who need it. If you are sensitive at all, if you feel the lash of the suffering of others on your back, this panorama of life and strength denied is like remaining helpless while the hands of the drowning are stretched toward you out of the water, is like listening, powerless, to the screams of those trapped in burning buildings.

Must we forget, harden ourselves against such sentiment? These are days of the triumph of death in human history. Can gentle sentiment now move the human mass? This after all is a civilization in which considerations of profit and loss are dominant, and there is no cost-accounting of mere bereavement, heartbreak caused by human erosion. Out with sentiment, then? Realists, it is the appalling waste of human energy that must concern us. It is the pouring down the rat hole of vast amounts of wealth—measurable!—that should engage our attention. This can be checked by competent use of known forces for human conservation. Is it too much to hope that political leaders can be made to understand this: That if communicable disease is wiped out, and curable disease controlled, then we could plug up the drain on the nation's treasury due to present perpetuation of preventable and controllable illness and death?

IV

The causes of the time lag between the discovery of science and its human use are complicated. Yet they can be spotted, broken down into their simple elements, and largely liquidated. Every community is responsible; each locality can take part, yet the fight cannot be effectively started without a nation-wide program of human conservation. The following facts are not debatable. The health services of the nation are grossly inadequate. Its hospital, laboratory, and health center facilities are nonexistent in wide areas, and are miserably under-financed in others. A formidable proportion of the nation's people who have small incomes or no incomes, get not enough medical service, or poor medical service, or no medical service at all. This is no mere New Deal viewing with alarm. These facts have been accepted in principle by the House of Delegates, the governing body of the American Medical Association. They are more than facts in principle. They are facts, indisputable.

Less than a third of our counties, and an even smaller proportion of our cities, have full-time trained health officers. This means that the doctors, the soldiers who fight sickness and death, are operating without a general staff on two thirds of the sectors of the health front.

Great areas of our country—especially rural ones —are totally without the services of nurses. There is no city in the country in which nursing—public health and general—can be called adequate.

Vast regions—again especially rural ones—are devoid of general hospitals, hospital-health-centers with modern laboratories which are the strong points of a modern war against sickness and death.

To keep the people of our nation healthy and able to earn their livings to produce the nation's wealth, the average level of the budgets of our state health departments is at the miserable figure of 11 cents *per capita*. It is profitable to ponder this, at the same time remembering that the cost of merely hospitalizing the consumptives of a city like Detroit is more than one dollar *per capita* of all of its citizens annually.

There is no need of an expensive nationwide survey preliminary to organizing a national health program. Our healthmen and doctors know what deaths can be wiped out, what sickness controlled by now known science. They know where mass tragedy and waste of human life is greatest; they know the hot spots of misery and death. The physicians, laboratory workers, and potential healthmen exist and can be quickly trained into an effective force for human conservation. Our university medical schools—underfinanced though they are—already turn out the most competent body of young doctors, medical scientists, and healthmen in the world. It is true that if medical science were to be turned on full power, more physicians, laboratorians, nurses, and healthmen than now exist would be needed. Yet enough exist to make a beginning.

But this is the stymie: no nationwide program can be organized without the help of the federal government. It is true that local and state governments could profitably implement local human conservation if they would put up the money. But you cannot get blood out of a stone. It is a fact that many counties, cities, states, have not the financial resources to fight a truly powerful war against death. The deterioration, the human erosion of one part of our country, is a drain on all of it. The nation is now trying to fight unemployment, bad housing, low wages nationally. And we can ask, with Doctor Thomas Parran, why these should be made national programs, while we leave to forces of laissez faire the problem of the sickness of the people? For it is basic that bad health contributes to these other factors now swelling the army of the dependent. Sickness strikes down millions of otherwise self-supporting persons. Human erosion is a major cause of poverty and destitution. And these are prime causes of the relief burden—which whether we like it or not must remain, much of it, national.

There is no question that local doctors and healthmen should fight their own local war against sickness and death in their own local regions. But in many states, cities, counties, they cannot begin without federal help. Why is this just principle of federal grant in aid—which has worked well in our highway development—called in question when our most competent men against death wish to apply it to fight for life?

And yet, without such financial help, without technical advice by the U. S. Public Health Service, a national program of human conservation has little or no chance of getting started.

The above story of human erosion was published

in *Country Gentleman* for March, 1939. The outline of now possible human conservation was published in the April issue, and is now presented in a more detailed form, but with no departure from the essence of the argument.

III. Human Conservation *

THIS IS now the grave question: Do those raising this or that objection to a national health program really want to begin possible action against human erosion? The objections raised have been based upon bogeys of regimentation of doctors, or upon technical difficulties in administration of the federal moneys needed.

Yet there is growing hope for human conservation. The viewers with alarm, the technical objectors—though in high positions of power—are few in numbers. And they are nervous about the discontent of the people.

There are signs that they are beginning to feel the rising ground swell of popular indignation over needless sickness and death. Maybe the people's anger is not yet strong enough to precipitate national action for a health law tomorrow. Maybe, as Thomas Parran suggests, popular pressure is still feeble because

* Substantially as printed in *Country Gentleman*, April 1939.

"'it is always the other fellow who is apt to be sick."
But only maybe.

Because there is evidence, too, that the people are
not so completely selfish, egotistical. There are signs
that they consider not only themselves, but feel the
lash of the suffering of others upon their own backs.
In the popular poll by the American Institute of
Public Opinion—1937—they gave within a few per
cent of a unanimous YES—to the question of whether
the federal government should expend twenty-five
million dollars a year to fight syphilis.

—Yet no estimable citizen expects, himself, to
contract this shameful sickness—

And again, the menace and shame of this blood
taint to others, to the nation, were so great that popular pressure forced a unanimous vote of YES for a
Venereal Disease Control Act through both houses
of Congress. And it is not the fault of the people, or
of Congress, that the moneys authorized have not
been appropriated. . . .

And yet, even though altruism for public health
is on the upsurge, it is here acknowledged that the
personal question—Why should I be needlessly sick,
why should I needlessly die?—is still the most
powerful ferment among the people for public health
action. And here the already enormous and always

growing public demand for news and more news—
from newspapers, popular magazines, radio—about
medical discoveries is making this portentous question more real, more bitter to the mass of the people.
More and more, you, and you, and you, realize—

That you may walk, a little weak in the knees, out
of your doctor's office. You have just been told you
must have a grave operation. Cancer is not mentioned, only hinted, but delicately. And you know
that you live in one of those great areas of our country where the doctors do not have the scientific training or the laboratory equipment to say surely yes or
no about that possible cancer. Where doctors do not
have the high training or technical weapons to save
you even if they do find your peril in time.

You realize you live in one of those regions where
medical science is not instantly available to meet the
deadly emergency of pneumonia. This is third in
rank of the master killers which now could be made
next to negligible by serums and sulfapyridine!
These are weapons that may not be for you because
the training to use them and the laboratories to guide
their use have not been supplied to your doctor.

You realize too that childbirth has at last become
a public health question, that it is no longer a matter
of the physician's discretion whether a mother shall

live or die. But you may know that you inhabit a city, village, or county where death's batting average against childbearing women remains scandalously high. Or where unscientific obstetrical care, if it does not kill your wife, may result in her life-wreck.

You have it driven home to you, too, that among your neighbors—if you are unlucky enough to live in the wrong community—there is heartbreak shattering the hoped-for joy of parenthood. There is grief over children stillborn, or blind, or maimed and spastic, or imbecile, or living healthy for a few days only then to die. And the needlessness of this butchery, this maiming at life's beginning, is becoming a bitter thing to millions, and to you.

You begin to ponder—though impressed by the hurrah about the conquest (?) of consumption—over the fact that there still remain some four hundred thousand actively tuberculous sick, spewing death about the nation. You ask whether there really is a special guardian angel hovering to guard your own children from this white death.

You may comfort yourself, saying: There's no insanity in *our* family. You hope that your children belong among the lucky nineteen out of every twenty who may not have to be put in a mental institution during the coming years. But you realize that there is still argument over whether most forms of insanity do "run in families." Your own child may not then be exempt from the menace of mental sickness. And you have been told that, in your own state, the physicians have not the wherewithal to use the new marvelous weapons just discovered for the cure of mental disease.

You are in the prime of life, you are riding the crest. Sudden heart-wreck, ruined kidneys, brain stroke—these are not for you. But yesterday your equally robust friend was stricken. In your community where there may be opportunity—but only for the lucky minority—to take advantage of careful periodic examinations by highly trained physicians with all laboratory tests available. Had this science been available for all, your friend might be now alive with a longer lease on active life.

Millions of Americans are mulling over this, they are beginning to mutter their disgust about this grim fact: that, by the law of averages, one or another of these more or less preventable perils may tomorrow reach out—for themselves. By newspapers, magazines, radio they are informed that the defeat of these dangers could begin now. They begin to murmur, asking—

Why, when the more fortunate among us can take

out insurance to put bread into the mouths of our families, roofs over their heads, clothing on their bodies, learning into their brains—

And why, when there is vast promise of these fundamentals as human rights, regardless of economic level—

Then why must there be delay, buck-passing, economic and technical objection to a national program for human conservation—to insure not mere medical care but longer, stronger, happier life, for us, for our own?

II

It is characteristic of a primitive civilization such as our own—where democracy means that you may shoot off your mouth about anything but does not yet mean that you have a right to life—it is natural that action for human conservation must grow out of argument. All health planners—practical or crackpot—will have and are now having their say. Can a practical program for human conservation be distilled out of the present welter of proposals? How fast can we go, and down what roads, to give more power to our men of medicine and our public healthmen who do not technically object, who are not afraid, who believe they can now begin to expand the fight for life?

There is news that legislation is about to be proposed by Senator Wagner—to spend vast sums of money for medical care. Publisher Frank Gannett and a medical cohort are getting ready to fight it. But Senator Wagner's health bill—this is January, 1939—will undoubtedly have the inside track. Can Congress, on the other hand, be prevailed upon to consider a sane plan for human conservation, essentially non-controversial, beginning without the throwing about of vast sums of money or the setting up of an army of jobholders?

Such a plan does exist. It is in process of development by a small and entirely informal group of new men against death. It aims at the enlistment—in a volunteer health army not regimented into government jobs—of the nation's physicians, nurses, laboratorians, engineers, healthmen. The plan has limited, yes, modest objectives. Its primary aim is a nation-wide attack upon sickness and death rates. Its purpose is to cut these down by concerted effort against all now preventable, or partially controllable, or curable disease and death.

This program plays no favorites among the people. It is to strike at the sickness and death rates of all classes and levels of all the people—without regard to their religion, their color, their virtues or faults, or their power to pay for this science.

This plan probably has psychological short-comings. Its concentration upon sickness and death-rate curves makes it seem heartless, maybe, like an engineer's blueprint. Its statement that the fight for human conservation should be a fight against waste of national wealth—this may make it a bit dull, like a business balance sheet.

—Yet it sold well to the people of Detroit—in the economic fight against tuberculosis—

But can our healthmen, scientists, doctors—they are all too human—nerve themselves to this mathematical, this cost-accounting slant at the inherently emotional question of living or dying?

—Yet emotional appeals have not given them adequate weapons to fight heartbreak and bereavement—

But the plan demands a new slant, a new mental and emotional fusion. Physicians must keep, as ever, their focus upon the healing and the good health of the individual sick man, woman, child. Yet they are going to have to join with the healthmen, biologists, actuarial experts, engineers, in a march toward a goal that is arithmetical, that is surely remote, possibly unattainable—reaching, as they are going to have to, toward the final eradication of all preventable sickness and death. The generalissimo of this projected adventure in human conservation is no human being, really. The boss of the project is the downing of the sickness and death rates. To the undoubted fears that this is inhuman, heartless, this can be answered—

Mass medical care, personal medical care will not be neglected but intensified under this plan. Without the best medical care all projects of disease prevention must fail. And allowing people to remain sick of diseases not yet preventable but already curable—that would be an indefensible drain upon the nation's resources under the proposed economic health program.

Here, substantially and specifically, are the aims of this proposed economic plan of human conservation—

Our new men against death believe: That they could drive tuberculosis down toward negligible in little more than a generation. That they could wipe out malaria in a dozen or fifteen years. That before your own babies have grown to man- or womanhood, the danger of syphilis could be made a vanishing one. That your daughter's chance of death or permanent life-wreck from childbirth could be cut down two-thirds. That the chance that her babies could be born living and then remain alive and healthy could be doubled. That if you're young today, your chance to die from cancer could be made a third less than it is now. That pneumonia—third ranking killer—could be cut down to the now relative impotence of diphtheria. And as for insanity, within a generation the walls of our asylums would no longer be bulging with daft ones, and the keepers might be looking round for inmates to fill up their beds and thrash round in their padded cells. . . .

These are the hopes and even the promises of our new men against death, provided—

Provided that our political leaders would let them give their science full gun, let them direct its use, full power.

Provided there is active, whole-hearted co-operation from the doctors of the nation.

These promises are based upon now known science. And with discoveries constantly now being made in our laboratories, and with the greater blooming of discovery that would follow the program's encouragement of medical research and education, these now predictable triumphs would be far surpassed at the end of a generation. . . .

III

These, you say, are strong words, tall promises. Yet this campaign for human conservation contemplates nothing revolutionary in science or in human relations. It means, simply, the encouragement, the speeding up of a closer relation between doctors and public healthmen that has been developing—with no hurrah and not much medical opposition—during the past two generations. During the past forty years there has been an at first hesitant and suspicious, but gradually closer and more cordial teamwork against death—by doctors, healthmen, laboratorians, engineers, nurses. The national program of human conservation would require only that this teamwork be—intensified.

Already there has been forty years of work to down sickness and death rates. Has the bleak arithmetic of this objective taken the heart and enthusiasm out of these still primitive teams of fighters for life? On the contrary. But you protest that politicians—since they are notoriously baby-kissers, not economists—could never be led to support public health expansion on the cold proposition that public health expansion would save the nation money. You say that all politicians *talk* money saving, but never act as if they understood its necessity. Yet the opposite—by certain local politicians—has already been locally demonstrated.

In Michigan, laboratory and public healthmen—co-working with the state's practicing physicians—have cut down the state's diphtheria death rate from 25.2 per 100,000 population in 1920 to 1.4 in 1937.

Who gave them the sinews of war to do this? The toxoid preventive—the State Laboratories produce enough of it for all Michigan's children—demands an annual outlay of $35,000. By mass protection of Michigan's children, toxoid has wiped out an annual diphtheria hospital bill of more than $500,000. But what politician would understand this simple bookkeeping, or would have the intelligence to believe in the promise of a man of medical science that this saving could be effected?

The money needed for the state's manufacture of the diphtheria toxoid, for distributing it—free—to all Michigan's physicians, was appropriated by Governor Alex Groesbeck and the state legislators. This was done by these politicians upon the demonstration, by Doctor C. C. Young, Director of the State Laboratories, that this expenditure would save the state money.

Not lives, or lives only as a by-product!

Against syphilis—and by a like economic device—
the physicians of the state of Wisconsin have won
a like stunning victory. In 1916, out of every one
hundred first admissions to the state's asylums, thirteen came, stricken with the final consequence of
syphilis, paresis. Doctor William F. Lorenz prevailed upon the state fathers to appropriate a modest
sum of money to his Wisconsin Psychiatric Institute.
So that he could offer free blood tests, to be taken by
Wisconsin's practicing physicians upon all of their
patients—whether or no syphilis was suspected.

That was in 1916. The doctors found a vast
amount of unsuspected syphilis. They treated it. By
1937 they had cut down the tragic parade of paretics
into the state's mental hospitals from the old high
of thirteen per one hundred first admissions to four
per one hundred.

The blood test was free to the doctors. It costs the
state five cents per test. While it costs the state $2000
to maintain each paretic in hospital till death relieves
him of his dreadful stigma. The doctors increased
their practices. Thousands of people—otherwise
marked for imbecile death—are now working because their syphilis was detected in time. They support their families, which otherwise would have

likely been added to Wisconsin's relief load. They add to the wealth of Wisconsin. Syphilis is now actually so rare in Wisconsin that medical professors find it hard to find typical cases to show their students.

Then why a national health program? If individual states can win such individual death fights, why can't all health programs against all preventable disease be organized, and fought, locally? The majority of the states, cities, counties—and this includes the relatively rich ones—have not the financial power for a fight on all sectors of the battle against death. Michigan, triumphant over diphtheria, goes on being syphilitic because there is lack of syphilis-fighting money. Wisconsin, victorious over syphilis, seems not to be able to find the wherewithal for a really adequate fight against tuberculosis.

Yet a question arises here. It is an embarrassing one. It must be laid upon the doorstep of our men of medical science, our physicians, our public healthmen. Individuals, far-seeing men of the future like Cy Young in Michigan, Bill Lorenz in Wisconsin, Henry Vaughan in the city of Detroit, these and others have been able to get driblets of death-fighting money from politicians, and have then demonstrated the enormous money-saving—we say nothing of life-saving—that resulted. But there they have stopped. They have not gone the next simple step farther. They have not said, Mr. Governor, Mr. Mayor, Mr. Representative, Mr. Senator—we have saved you, we have saved the citizens, the taxpayers, these millions. Are you not going to put a part of these savings to our credit, for our laboratories, our hospitals, for the further fight of our men against death? Will you kindly call in your auditors? Will you see that they credit us—your men against death—with the money, it's millions, we've already saved you? Will you then base your public health appropriations on this cost-accounting? Will you allow us a fair fraction of this profit? To plow back into our money- and life-saving business?

What would the voters do to their politicians who refused to act upon this demonstration of public health economy?

But this must be faced about our men against death: they are over-modest. They too easily get the wind up when they get their budgets from political magnificoes. They have not yet learned to by-pass these job-holders. By use of the newspapers and radio, they can now go straight to the people, showing them how their political leaders are not only neglectful of human life, but economically wasteful

when, in a lordly manner, they dole out their financial crumbs to the public health Lazaruses. Our men
against death do not yet realize how high they are
in public esteem. When they do realize it, act upon
it, then maybe local financing of human conservation
—even in poor communities—can be put upon a business basis.

There's another obstacle to the complete financing
of local death fights without some government aid.
The finances in communities, the policies of communities, are in general not long range. The finances
are not in general set up so that it is possible to spend
nickels today to save dollars twenty years hence.
Take Detroit. In its TB fight, the city fathers agreed
that the additional yearly appropriation of $200,000
to Henry Vaughan's health department budget,
would, in the future, save the city many millions of
dollars. But the city's charter empowered them to
appropriate this money for one year only. The whole
project is then at the mercy of future ignorant
mayors, aldermen who'd pinch pennies now, and
devil take the future.

How can any continuous effective human conservation project be carried on under conditions so "iffy"?

The federal government, on the other hand—
though it too sets up annual budgets—has more

power to finance long-range projects, such as those of defense, and conservation of natural resources. Is the conservation of human life a lesser question?

And will the people by and by begin to ask whether in the matter of living or dying, we are one nation, or again a house divided? The TB and syphilis microbes murdering Mississippi planters are the same that sap the strength of Ohio industrial workers, the same from which the rich are now largely exempt. The tubercle and syphilis microbes know nothing about state boundaries. They are only fought in regions and among people that can afford to fight them. Can our country long exist, can it realize its possible future greatness, half sick and half strong? Today there is a criminal spottiness about the fight for life. Healthwise we are not a house united.

IV

The people themselves, only awaiting leaders, are ready to come to the aid of those fighters for life who will soon be regarded as the first citizens of the nation. The people would even now vote the sinews of war demanded by human conservation. The voters must first of all know how our new men against death propose to begin their battle. In the first place, there is no need to set up a vast public health or medical bureaucracy. It is proposed only to mobilize our physicians, nurses, public healthmen, engineers, scientists into a volunteer, not rigidly regimented, army. The war against sickness and death would be under local control. A state authority would supervise it. Federal authority would lead, advise, and help to finance it. The U. S. Public Health Service is ready now—and it is the one federal agency competent to do this—to expand its advisory expert services. It will supervise the proposed federal grants in aid to the states, to each according to their needs. It will help those states poorest and most backward, to educate adequate death-fighting personnel, to build the laboratories, health centers, hospitals needed. In the more prosperous states, too, the death fight will be intensified. Each local health program will be advised, supervised, in turn by the state health authority—representatives of the physicians of the state co-working with state health and welfare agencies. The front line fight—in each community—will be entrusted to the local physicians and healthmen. They will be aided in every way to raise local medical and public health competence, to build the needed laboratories, health centers, hospitals.

Dominating the entire program would be the prevention of sickness and death. Our new men against death do not consider schemes of national compulsory health insurance. Those would demand a new formidable bureaucracy. They would turn the doctors into job-holders, and whether or not it would be good for the doctors, the doctors bitterly resent this. Compulsory health insurance schemes make provision for a great expansion in *quantity* of medical care. They do not provide for better quality of the care of the sick. And, finally, compulsory health insurance is really sickness insurance. It assumes the continuance of sickness. It does not recognize the prime duty of our death fighters to eliminate preventable death and disease. Basil O'Connor, practical layman, illuminates this question by an excellent illustration. We are all concerned over the national scandal of traffic death and injury, he says. But we would not for one moment think that the *principal* weapon against motor accidents is compulsory motor accident insurance. The chief weapons are the building of accident-proof highways, the training of drivers, the constantly improved motor-car safety devices, and the policing of reckless drivers. Alfred Harcourt, equally practical, asks how can a rural community best cut down its excessive fire insurance rates? Of course by equipping and maintaining a well-manned fire department.

So with the conservation of human health and life. A vast proportion of America's sickness, that would demand enormous compulsory insurance payments, is preventable, eradicable. Compulsory health insurance is locking the door after the horse has left the barn. Why not wipe out this preventable sickness and save the bulk of this proposed vast amount of insurance money?

Yet the cost of medical care—today—is an insupportable burden to the majority of our citizens. But the charity work demanded of our doctors to give the people the inadequate medical care they now get, is also a burden to the doctors. And all over the country the physicians are beginning to realize this. If certain of their own medico-political leaders are complacent about the state of our medical care, many of the rank-and-file physicians, and the vast majority of the real medical leaders, are restive. And the physicians themselves are best qualified to organize the voluntary group medical service plans that will justly spread the present insupportable burden of people in the low and moderate income brackets.

What elimination of our national human erosion calls for is not state medicine, but good medicine, modern medicine—but available to every far-flung community and practiced in the American manner. In lonely farmhouses, in hovels and tenements of the underdog millions, in the homes of the middle class, in hospitals, it's the family doctor who first sees sick folks. Sick or well, for a long time into the future, the American people are going to pick their own doctor. Any human conservation program that tried overnight to change this ingrained custom would collapse before it got started.

Yet, we must face it: the new discipline of applying modern science to the death fight is going to be a stern one. It demands continual scientific training, constant refreshing of medical and public health knowledge on the part of our physicians, healthmen, laboratorians. For this there is now no general provision. As famed Harvard surgeon Elliott C. Cutler points out, most doctors practice what they learned in medical school. And for that reason medical practice is, as a rule, from fifteen to twenty-five years behind the knowledge available in the centers of medical learning and research, in the medical schools and universities. . . .

The program of human conservation proposed by our new men against death demands a new kind of death fighter. It requires a highly skilled army of doctors, trained to use the delicate tests of diagnosis, the powerful but two-edged curative and preventive weapons that can now cut down, control, wipe out today's sickness and death rates from pneumonia, syphilis, malaria, insanity, cancer, maternal and infant mortality. These scientific tools have been developed, most of them, in the past dozen years. They are being improved constantly by medical research. To ask our rank-and-file doctors out of school for a dozen years and more to use these weapons without training, is as silly as it would be to man modern anti-aircraft cannon with minute-men of '76 who had learned to blaze away with nothing more modern than a muzzle-loading musket.

This must be admitted: that the great army of doctors who will volunteer for the new human conservation program, must be paid for the time they will have to take off from their practices to learn to use the new death-fighting weapons.

This must be acknowledged: that medicine as today practiced remains too much a horse-and-buggy, pill-prescribing, let-us-see-your-tongue business. Too few doctors realize that the laboratory has become the heart of the modern fight against human erosion. The daily, the routine, the incessant use of the laboratory will have to be made available to our doctors, rural as well as urban, and the need to use the laboratory will have to be taught them, brought home to them. The life-guarding power of today's delicate blood and tissue examinations, x-rays, chemicals, serums and vaccines, can only begin its cutting down of sickness and death if all of the nation's physicians understand how to use some, and appreciate the importance of all, of these weapons.

And, in addition to constant training in these new skills, in the use of them, another education of physicians is demanded by a program of human conservation. Though there are hopeful signs that many physicians are beginning to feel the lash of suffering on the backs of other people, yet some conduct their practices as if they were running luxury shops on Fifth Avenue in New York City. For these medical die-hards, life, strength, is for those who can pay for it. Books could and should be written telling true stories of this ignorant point of view. Human conservation—nationwide—cannot be developed till the nation's doctors as a profession act upon this basic principle—

That all the patients of every doctor will have full benefit of the new powerful science—

Regardless of the amount of money in the pocket of any man, woman, or child.

V

Just as it would be idiotic to send an army to war without modern mechanized weapons, so it would be silly to expect our human conservation fight to be started without nationwide ample technical equipment, without proper modern laboratories and hospitals. The enthusiasm with which our nation's high political command recommends appropriations of billions for the army and navy, while it remains niggardly toward the medical and health needs of the people this army and navy is supposed to defend—this contrast is today's most ghastly humor.

The lacks of laboratories and hospitals are already mapped. A building program for health centers and hospitals, and help in the improvement and maintenance of excellent hospitals already existing—these are essential preliminaries to the proposed fight against human erosion. Here and there over the nation, thousands on the waiting lists of TB sanatoria rot to death with consumption. Scores of thousands remain daft because of the totally inadequate organization for modern treatment of the mentally sick. General hospitals, not adequately equipped and staffed to diagnose early cancer and cure it, turn scores of thousands of cancer sufferers away—because it is too expensive for these penny-pinched institutions to house such poor people while they are dying. We point with pride to our existing handsome hospital piles of brick and mortar. They are a mockery, a national shame, if they cannot offer their healing, their relief of suffering, to all Americans—regardless.

But there are wide regions of our country where the citizens cannot even console themselves with this tragi-comedy of existing hospitals that cannot afford to house them for their healing or soothing of pain. National human conservation requires that, in such regions, hospital-laboratory health centers be built. These will be the strong points in today's no-man's land of the fight for life. They are lacking in many cities. They are almost nonexistent in vast rural areas where the practice of preventive and curative medicine is now hardly more than medieval.

If we, as citizens, could only lay our hands on a modest bit of that always available tank and battleship money, the building of these strong-points for life could soon begin. Each would house a modern laboratory, manned by laboratorians—of whom there are not now enough, but who could be found from among the ranks of our young physicians and trained for this purpose. These hospitals would be run by local physicians. They would give our doctors the science to spot and fight preventable death, all preventable death—from the hemorrhage of a new-born babe to the cancer of old men and women. Here would be x-ray apparatus, blood-grouping and blood-transfusion machinery, oxygen appliances, electrocardiographs, metabolism machines. Here would be medical consultants to co-work and advise with family physicians, to establish—informally—that practice of medicine by groups of specialists which without doubt is the medicine of the future. Here would be libraries where doctors could keep abreast of modern death-fighting science; and physicians enlisted in the human conservation program would be ashamed not to do so.

Finally, to exert their full power for human conservation, these hospital health centers could be life-saving lighthouses for the people. They could be rallying points, meeting places for parents, young people, children. Here by lectures our doctors could tell the citizens the stirring stories of how science can now build their strength. Here by movies like "The Fight for Life" of Film Director Pare Lorentz, young and old would be gripped and stirred by the promise of medical science in a world now dedicated to blood and death.

And just as our doctors are beginning to abandon the secrecy, the mystery, of their ancient ethics, just as the best ones among them are becoming life-teachers and guides for the people, so the people can teach their own needs to healthmen and doctors—

For the physicians still underestimate popular intelligence. Figure to yourself such a people's health forum in the meeting hall of one of the new hospital-health centers. Here farmers and their wives, businessmen and workmen could meet, asking their doctors—

Why aren't you allowed to x-ray our whole community, every citizen, to spot all early tuberculosis?

Why doesn't everybody in the community—preachers included—get a periodic blood test for syphilis?

Why isn't our county laboratory man investigating this new horse sickness? It may be encephalitis. It might jump to our children.

What's wrong with the new whooping-cough vaccine? It made Mrs. Smith's baby mighty sick.

Our county has had eight maternal deaths this year. How come?

Farmer Jones has a bad x-ray burn from his cancer treatment. Does his doctor know how to use these new deep x-rays?

Why did Mr. Brown—he was a mighty good citizen—have to die of pneumonia? He didn't get sulfapyridine till he'd been sick four days.

It is to the people that the proposed new army of human conservation will be responsible. The physicians, nurses, healthmen, will be exactly as competent as its boss, the people, demands.

V I

Of course our political leaders will meet the demand for a program of human conservation with this time-honored out, this alibi—

"But where are we going to get the money?"

It is a powerful, a murderous, little question. It mocks the people who want to live. It confuses the federal, state, municipal, and county healthmen eager to begin the battle. It gives excellent excuse for delay to medical die-hards who maintain that no national health program is necessary in this so-healthy America. It baffles the growing army of still voiceless physicians who want to be co-workers for human conservation. This nasty little question, an up till now all-powerful negation of the right to live, has its allies in those who really hold the financial power of the nation. In the bankers.

But these, too, are human, and believe it or not, when you get to know them, they do not relish their ill fame as blood-suckers, parasites, inhibitors of the potential productive power of the nation. Aren't there some among them who could be enlisted in the ranks of our new men against death? Their job is now to audit, to account for, to conserve the nation's money wealth, and to use that wealth in expanding the nation's productive power. But couldn't our financiers give the answer to that deadly little question of where we are to get the money? So doing, they could lead the new health army into action.

The bankers are the only existing experts able to draw up a new kind of balance sheet. They could show the President, the Congress, how with adequate and modest funds our men against death could change the red ink of today's human erosion to the black ink of tomorrow's human conservation. The bankers could point out to our political leaders the terrific cost, the scandalous wastefulness, the burden on the tax-payers and on the financial stability of communities, that results from allowing this mass human erosion to go on.

The bankers could use one little example, showing our treasury's watchdogs the frightful cost of maintaining one disease, dementia praecox. Horatio M. Pollock, Director of Mental Hygiene Statistics for the State of New York, has estimated the burden of this form of insanity on our country. The money cost of the mere hospital care of these unfortunate hundreds of thousands he calculates to be approximately $100,000,000 a year. He estimates, further, that the economic loss due to their disability and premature death amounts to $175,000,000 annually. The total money loss of this one disease adds up to $275,000,000. This shame could now begin to be strikingly reduced by a moderate amount of millions making possible the modern curative treatment of this mental sickness. But to maintain this infamy *our country pours out, in hard cash in two years, more than the total cost of building the Panama Canal.*

This is the loss due to one single sickness. What would the total money loss of human erosion amount to if our death-fighting bankers would turn their accountants and actuarial hounds loose on syphilis, pneumonia, tuberculosis, cancer, heart disease, and the various forms of rheumatism?

These sums—accurate—would reach an astronomic total annually. Our bankers could set out this red ink of the gigantic deficit due to sickness, death, deterioration, running into billions of dollars yearly.

Projecting this red ink balance sheet on the screen, they could then say, respectfully, to the President, to Congress—

How can you say there is no available money? Isn't it short-sighted to give the people this alibi for failure to provide the modest number of millions that would set a program of human conservation going? You say, Mr. President, Mr. Congress, that there's no available money because vast sums now have to be spent for unemployment, for social security? But a powerful program of human conservation will save a vast part of this expenditure. And it will prevent spending of greater sums that you are going to have to pour out—to keep alive, no, half alive, the millions of citizens who are not sound, energetic, resourceful human animals—which medical science could make them. Do you not understand that here is a prime cause of that very social insecurity you now struggle to ameliorate—

Millions of our people, needlessly deteriorated, feeble in energy, cannot weather the economic storms they would laugh at if they were healthy and strong.

Becoming biologists for the moment, our bankers would point out that the poverty of our out-of-joint economic system helps to cause half-living human bodies, dull brains, feeble hands. But they know the opposite, too: the strong hands and alert brains that science could build would give us more Americans who would not long tolerate our joblessness, our economic enfeeblement.

—Surely we cannot believe that our political eleemosynars, the present dolers-out of our so-called social security, wish to perpetuate a half-alive America? To perpetuate their own political power?—

So at last our bankers could once and for all turn to public ridicule that up-till-now unanswerable question of where do we get the money.

Traditionally our money masters have been held to be enemies of human kindness, largely devoid of human sentiment. They themselves are today shaken. They are in despair of the health of that system which, so potent in developing means of production, seems now unable to distribute what it can make. . . . Yet sensible people—disillusioned as they now must be about socialism's promises—realize that our American way, while not so hot, is all we've got to keep us together, to keep us going as a nation. But new vigor could be put into our present sick system. If, joining the fight for human conservation, using their great skill and experience in the development of a new kind of economy, our bankers would take the lead in the fight against human erosion.

They are not heartless, they do not yet realize, they haven't it burned into them that death does not wait. Hasn't the hour struck for them to join the new men against death, to come on the march with public-spirited physicians, healthmen, scientists? Holders of the nation's purse strings, they must be listened to by political leaders.

Is it not up to our financiers to join the people in asking the President, the Congress, to permit the beginning of a nation-wide fight for human energy, human life—a war based on the one consideration about which so much is said and so little done. Based on economy.

Of course it may be asked whether our bankers are free agents to suggest this economic health program? Are our bankers now more than cogs in the U. S. Treasury set-up?

IV. The Fifth Human Right

THESE STORIES of *Human Erosion* and *Human Conservation* were delivered to Philip Rose for publication, in the Winter of 1939. And 1939 began with a stir of hope that a practical national health program might be enacted into law. There was hope of it, certainly, among those large pressure groups of the people who remembered the surge of enthusiasm for health, any kind of health plan, the more money for health the merrier, at Miss Roche's health conference in July, 1938. There was hope among a few of the new men against death, still ignorant of political mysteries. Editor Phil Rose, though cagy and skeptical of politicians as always, was encouraging. He had not thought the foregoing denunciation of the infamy of human erosion too bitter to print in his fireside farmpaper. He approved the foregoing plan for human conservation and prepared to publish it. Anything but a New Dealer, Rose didn't believe a plan so non-controversial would be blocked by politics—if only it could be got before Congress.

"There may be a few hard-shelled anti-Administration people who would block anything, however good, that the New Deal proposes," Rose said. "In fact I am sure there are such hard-shelled crustaceans."

—Remember, no part of what's called the New Deal had yet approved the human conservation program—

But the people? "The great mass of the American people," said Rose, "want to live. They don't give a tinker's damn which or whose political party is in power. They want a good America."

So this mass magazine editor believed here was a question over which politics could be adjourned. And his company, Rose felt sure, would wholeheartedly approve the proposed health program. Should we simply print these stories in the *Country Gentleman*, call it a day, consider them bread thrown on the waters? No. They were pamphleteering, said Rose, and that means action. But how to try to get it? We had no pressure group, no lobby at all. Our foray toward the high political command in 1938 had been a flop. What now to do? Was it time now? You know—timing is everything. . . .

What our new men against death were after, of course, was the establishment of the first human right, declared in 1776 to be self-evident by the founding fathers. Only our moderns were modest, not demanding that this right to life should have first place. When in 1776 the founding fathers wrote that beautiful thought, they were being—literary. In those days—pre-medical science—the right to life was at the disposal of God, not man. It is only since Pasteur, since Koch, since the rise of the microbe hunters and men against death of the past two most wonderful generations in human record, that man himself dares to begin to dispose in the matter of life and death. But did our political leaders—with all due respect—understand the mighty new challenge, the dazzling hope of the new medical science?

Of course the President had gone on record. October 19, 1934, at Roanoke, Virginia, he had said: "I mentioned once upon a time that we must do first things first. The care of the disabled, the sick, the destitute and the starving in all ranks of our population—that, my friends, is the first thing."

Yet it had to be recognized as a fact that, since it had come to power, the New Deal in its battle for what is called "social security," had fought hardest for other rights than the right to life implied in the care of the sick and disabled. It had fought for the right to food, clothing, shelter, fuel. These had been its first four human rights. Was it ready now to fight for the fifth, the right to life itself, to that maximum of life as medical science, unchained, now has the power to give life and not mere existence to the people?

It seemed that this would be a shrewd move politically. Die-hards may argue against the rights of what they call our no-good shovel-leaning riffraff to eat well, to live in better than hovels, to dress warmly, to have a stick of wood or chunk of coal for the stove or fireplace. But it is rare to find a tory who, brought to the simple decision of live or die, would say die to the lowest sharecropper, the most forlorn gamin in the gutter.

"The health of the people is not controversial." But wasn't this platitude fooling our new men against death?

Wasn't this bad politics, bad timing? In a democracy can any great human right be won without controversy? After all, Lincoln had re-established the Union of States on the issue of the right of black people to liberty—but only after the awful controversy of the War of the Rebellion. Maybe this now possible right to life was not ready for action, for the very reason it had not become controversial. Maybe what was needed was the placing before the people of agitation against life for all. By to-day's worshipers of Nietzsche, Kaiser Wilhelm II, and Hitler. By those who today go on record as deny-ing life to all. By Mr. H. L. Mencken, who has recently written in *The Baltimore Sun*—

"There are backwaters of the South at this minute wherein the average intelligence of the country peo-ple, white and black alike, rises little if anything above that of an asylum for the feeble-minded. Cer-tainly it would be more sensible, and maybe more Christian to herd them into concentration camps, and there open up on them with bombs and artillery.

"They are completely useless, teetotally no good. . . .

"It is such simians . . . who are responsible for the rapid exhaustion of the natural resources of the United States [sic!] . . . This country can never be wholly civilized, and never more than half safe, until they are got rid of altogether."

For controversy, and to dramatize today's House Divided, if there were only more Menckens. If only hundreds of young Menckens—but brave—could go about the land, not from a safe chair in Baltimore recommending death to our underdogs, but flinging it in the teeth of millions of American citizens that for the good and the safety of their country, they should die. They could be promised death in an efficient American manner. Not by long Gestapo torture. Not by slow starvation, the horrible weapon of the crackpots of the Soviet Ogpu. But mercifully, by bombs and artillery. It would be feasible. The modern Samurai of the Christian Front could be recruited to realize Mr. Mencken's simple plan for his country's security.

Then the question of the right to life might well become controversial. Then again America would be a House Divided. Then we could have it out, have it over with. On the phoney issue of whether our land can exist, half blue-blood—half moron.

But away with irony. Nobody seriously hopes for the establishment of such an issue. The voice of Mencken has become a feeble one in the land for all its incitement to mass murder, its negation of life. The myrmidons that his cause would need, homicidal oafs and crackpots like those of the Christian Front, are bungling conspirators. Upon the question of human rights of all to shelter, food, health, there is now pretty general agreement. But there is lethargy. Is it because, maybe, out of our 130 millions not enough actually starve, or freeze to death, or are actually killed by lack of medical care? Is it because the nationwide disaster of human erosion is a hidden, diffused calamity going on in darkened rooms behind drawn curtains? Not dramatic like sudden mass dying by earthquake or flood. Is that why the people remain relatively apathetic about the right to health, because they are healthy—so-so? And because they can exist—so-so—they haven't the fire, the urge, to demand life stronger? It seems that this curious equilibrium has been reached in our country. This has, maybe, been established by the half use of medical science.

I I

So, failing the popular indignation needed to make the question of human conservation red hot politically, there was only one thing to try, and that was to make it red hot among our political leaders, among the high command of American politics. Here we were again, back where we began. Now the stories of human erosion, human conservation, in typescript and before they had been printed in Phil Rose's farm paper, were submitted to Basil O'Connor, friend of the President. Again as in the instance of that first little memorandum handed him the year before, Doc

O'Connor heartily approved these outlines of human erosion and its now possible combat.

"What's a more fundamental question?" Doc asked me. "What do we say to everybody when we first see them in the morning? We say, How are you? And how many answer it saying they feel fine? As a matter of fact most people you ask that, most of the time, feel lousy! That's what the title of these stories should be—How Are You? And shouldn't that be the first concern of the head of any nation?"

This was in Doc's best shrewd manner. And wasn't there hope, that if we only kept at him, the President would really begin to ask the nation, How are you? The new men against death were beginning to talk about health as a right, but hadn't the President gone on record, long ago, about the right of government to see to it that the governed had the right to life and health?

On June 25, 1929, at Saratoga Springs, New York, Governor Franklin Delano Roosevelt had said:

"Fifty years ago, the matter of health was individual; it was nobody's concern, except that of the family, whether a person was healthy or not, and gradually we have built up a new doctrine—the belief that the state has a positive right, not just an obligation, to see that the health of its individuals is brought up to a higher level."

Governor Roosevelt went even further, continuing: ". . . The old idea of the right of an individual to be sick or of a community to have epidemics no longer exists. That right has been turned around and transferred to the state."

This was heartening. This raised hopes.

So these statements of human erosion and its possible combat by a practical plan of human conservation started on their journey, it was hoped, to the White House. I waited and waited. Of their reception and their fate there came no word.

III

By now, early February, 1939, there was news that Senator Robert F. Wagner was about to introduce a health bill in the Congress. The President had transmitted the famous report of Miss Roche's Interdepartmental Committee to the Congress, not with a recommendation for action, but with advice that it be carefully studied. . . . This explains, without doubt, the Presidential silence on the statements regarding human erosion and conservation. After all Miss Roche's committee of government experts had been given that assignment. And who, indeed, were the members of our little modern "invisible college" of new men against death, to offer alternatives to the findings and projects of this Interdepartmental Committee?

Just the same, there was this to worry over. It was rumored that vast sums, reaching into figures of hundreds of millions of dollars yearly, were going to be recommended by the Wagner Bill, to implement a huge program of health and medical care. There was no hint that the program would be set up on the economic, self-liquidating basis that could satisfy Congressional budget-balancers. Shouldn't Senator Wagner be given the chance to look at a practical, a modest, a non-controversial health plan—which might bring budget-balancers and doctors alike along, and not antagonize them?

Howard Hunter now arranged an audience with Senator Wagner. For somewhat less than an hour that busy statesman sat, like a courteous and smiling Buddha, while the need of the economic viewpoint, the strong stressing of that viewpoint, was expounded to him. It was more than expounded, it was expostulated; and maybe this was my mistake, high-powering it too much, over-selling it? At any rate, the good Senator grinned pleasantly throughout, agreed in a sentence with the general principles put forward, asked me for copies of the human erosion and human conservation stories. These were furnished him, in typescript.

Of their fate nothing is known. Excepting that their influence on the Wagner Health Bill was nil.

Unhappy days were here again. From Detroit, from Health Commissioner Henry F. Vaughan, the father of the idea of an economic health plan, came bad news by wire. The Detroit TB fight, begun so gloriously on the recognition by the city fathers that it cost the city vast sums of money to let its citizens die of tuberculosis, that fight was now threatened with disaster. Now to New York came a wire from Henry Vaughan—

FIRST BUDGET SKIRMISH WITH MAYOR [RICHARD READING] REDUCES TUBERCULOSIS APPROPRIATION BY TWO THIRDS LEAVING APPROXIMATELY SIXTY-FIVE THOUSAND DOLLARS OUT OF TWO HUNDRED THOUSAND STOP DETROIT CITY GOVERNMENT ECONOMICALLY EMBARRASSED AND IT SEEMS APPARENT THAT LOCAL COMMUNITY CANNOT CARRY FULL EXPENSE OF ADEQUATE PREVENTIVE HEALTH PROGRAM STOP STRONGLY URGE FEDERAL AID TO CARRY ON TUBERCULOSIS PROGRAM WHICH HAS RESULTED IN UNCOVERING SEVEN HUNDRED THIRTY NEW CASES AND MADE

ESTIMATED SAVING IN HOSPITAL BILLS OF ONE MIL-
LION FIVE HUNDRED THOUSAND DOLLARS AT TWO
YEAR COST OF FOUR HUNDRED THOUSAND DOLLARS.

Here was documentary, yes, tragic evidence of the impotence of a community—even a powerful one like Detroit—to finance a death fight, even against one preventable sickness. If only men in the inner circles of high finance could hear this story. Mr. Harry L. Hopkins, now Secretary of Commerce, had appointed a business advisory council, including certain public-spirited financiers. An effort had been made to see Mr. Hopkins, an appointment had been arranged, but alas, the calendar of the Secretary of Commerce had become so full that the hoped-for interview was not granted.

There was an ace in the hole. There was a younger type of Wall Street financier that it was possible to reach. My friend, George D. Woods, Vice President of the First Boston Corporation, had studied the stories of human erosion and human conservation. He was enthusiastic. Woods is the type of banker who gives the lie to the libel that all money men are malefactors of great wealth. Woods, dealing in hundreds of millions, is himself not acquisitive. He is one of a new breed of cats in our economy, a sort of engineer, a technical man of high finance with no interest in the personal boodle levied by financial operators in the days of the robber barons. George Woods is a white hope for a re-birth of America's productive system. He does not forget that the sensible object of America's power to produce—is distribution. He does not go for Mr. Mencken's scheme of bombing underdogs. Now, having studied the outline for an economic plan for human conservation, Woods had an idea—

"Look," says George, "the American Investment Bankers' Association should go for this. We need to put forward something constructive for the country. We're in the dog house with the people, with the government, because we're always against everything. Now we're in the business of selling bonds of cities, states, communities. What's fundamental to the soundness of these securities? The financial soundness of the locality issuing the bonds, of course. And what's a major financial drain on every city, state, county? The big money drain of taking care of the needlessly sick. The money loss caused by heads of families dying—throwing their dependents on relief."

Why shouldn't the Investment Bankers' Association memorialize Congress, governors of states, mayors of cities, with these stories of human erosion and human conservation, accompanying them by a covering letter? It looked like a natural. A preliminary luncheon to a small group of investment bankers was given by Woods. They agreed—with one exception—to the soundness of the plan. But they objected that this, being urged by mere investment bankers, would carry no weight with the administration. The bankers, said they, were too much in the New Deal dog house.

So unhappier days were here again. The plan for pamphleteering action ended by the Curtis Publishing Company sending out marked copies of the *Country Gentleman,* carrying these stories, to all congressmen and senators.

But statesmen are busy, bedeviled by every kind of pressure group with a thousand different axes to grind. The response was negligible.

These were blue days in February, 1939, and, according to the personal discipline of never looking for an out, an alibi, I had to ask myself: What's wrong with the way those stories were written? Why didn't they click? Was the psychology wrong: talking of life and death in terms of dollars, and really meaning it? Had our success with that argument, in Detroit, been a fluke? Did anybody getting indignant about the money-waste of death really become more enthusiastic for life, more sentimental about it?

Yet in the gloom of that month of February, 1939, there was a gleam of hope. Doctor Ralph A. Fenton, of Portland, Oregon, member of the Board of Trustees of the American Medical Association, had read the economic human conservation program. He had approved it—"if it could be kept out of politics." Now through Doctor Fenton's kindness, this Board of Trustees, in Chicago, on February 17, 1939, in formal session, listened to a brief presentation of the plan. They were assured that—contrary to the belief of some of them—Doctor Thomas Parran was not committed to a scheme of national compulsory health insurance—the prevailing bugaboo of organized medicine. They were assured of Surgeon General Parran's eagerness to co-operate with the nation's doctors on some such plan as this economic health program. In fact he had been a co-planner with me, of this idea of human conservation. It was hinted to the Board of Trustees—and this was the idea of Basil O'Connor, close friend of the President—that if the American Medical Association and the national administration could be at the same time interested in our human conservation plan, there was a possibility of closing the rift between the New Deal and the doctors.

This was listened to with courtesy by the eminent physicians here assembled. It was kept in confidence, not spread on the minutes of the meeting. Copies of the stories of human erosion and conservation were sent to all the trustees, for their study and comment.

Then died this particular gleam of hope. It seemed as if every blow struck for human conservation was a blow aimed at something tangible, something solid, but always—as if in a bad dream—connecting with thin air.

And now the breach between the New Deal and the doctors was widening. High officials of the American Medical Association had been indicted by the Department of Justice. It was charged they had conspired with the District of Columbia Medical Society—in restraint of trade and did the doctors like their profession to be called a trade?—conspired to hinder certain Washington, D. C., physicians in their practice in a group medical plan. Now powerful personages in organized medicine were for fighting these indictments to the last ditch. There was promise of bitterness that would prevent co-operation toward a national health program between government and the doctors. And yet there was still a ray of hope. There were leading physicians who believed the health of the people would be best served if neither side—in what promised to be a legal dog-fight—should triumph.

Now the hubbub over the newly introduced S. 1620, the Wagner Health Bill, put an end to counsels of moderation, and certainly overshadowed the stories of human erosion and human conservation, just now published and distributed to America's rural millions. The Wagner Health Bill, like most New Deal measures, had a bad press. Senator Arthur Vandenberg keynoted against it. He was opposed, so he asserted, to any expansion of the government's social services "till we pay for those we have got." Quoting Michigan's favorite son with approval, the *Alliance* (Ohio) *Review* editorialized that, in its present state, the country could not afford to obligate itself to provide $80,000,000 next year, and $250,000,000 each year later on "to finance the latest New Deal effort to start an excursion into paternalism."

Apparently the Ohio editor thought the American people were in bouncing health. . . . That is the curious thing about the opening phases of the Wagner Bill controversy: that so little was said about the health of the people, excepting by its opponents, quoting the President himself, who said America's health was now better than it ever had been. . . .

There were sharp and just criticisms of the

Wagner Health Bill. Doctor Morris Fishbein—
quoted in an Associated Press release widely published—pointed out that it "would place control of
the health program in the hands of a few individuals. . . . Administration of it would be handled by
state health commissioners who would be answerable
only to the U. S. Public Health Service, the Social
Security Board, and the Department of Labor."

The inference—and it was a just one—was where
do the doctors come in, where do they get off
in this gigantic health program? Doctor Fishbein
might have gone further, asking what possible experience or competence have the Social Security Board
and the Department of Labor in public health and
medical care?

On the other hand, Doctor Fishbein omitted to
state the constructive fact that the U. S. Public
Health Service, provided it could be assured of the
co-operation of the country's doctors, was competent
to organize a health program and would co-operate
with the doctors.

Now in the *Charlotte* (North Carolina) *News*,
March 8, 1939, Doctor Fishbein was again quoted—

"Social Security doesn't change human nature or
create wealth. It merely enables the government to

try to do for the individual what he should have sense enough to do for himself."

Maybe so. But did this mean that the individual men, women, and children of the United States—and the doctors—could guard themselves against, could rid themselves of, the curse of tuberculosis, malaria, mental disease, pellagra, syphilis? Individually and without the help of local, state, and national health agencies? Come, come, Doctor!

Yet there is no question the Wagner Health Bill was a comedy of errors. And one of its weakest points was its accent on huge national spending, at the same time failing absolutely to set up machinery that would make health expenditure self-liquidating, that would show the people how a human conservation program—properly administered by federal, state, and local health agencies *and* the country's doctors—would pay for the original investment many times over.

To the antagonism of all but a few of the country's newspapers was now added the powerful voice of Publisher Frank Gannett. Aided by the ex-Kaiser's ex-propagandist, Doctor Edward Rumely, by health-man Haven Emerson, and by our advocate of bombing of human surplus underdogs—H. L. Mencken—

in a pamphlet the doctors of America were warned that they were in awful danger. Of regimentation.

In this hullabaloo what chance had a sane program aiming to raise the country's health level, to save the nation vast sums, by bringing the government and the physicians together? Yet there was a gleam of hope again. The Public Affairs Committee, in April, 1939, reprinted the *Country Gentleman's* stories of human erosion and human conservation. And here was the result: newspapers often critical of government spending were cordial to this economic health plan that so strongly accented national savings.

"In our preoccupation with questions of war and peace, of depression and unemployment, far too little attention has been given to the health of the people," editorialized the *Washington Post*. These stories of human erosion and human conservation "have rendered genuine service by re-emphasizing this critical need in clear and convincing terms. Their contribution will be especially appreciated in Washington, where an active fight for funds is going forward."

Best thanks to the *Post's* publisher, conservative but public-spirited Eugene Meyer. There was no evidence, however, of Mr. Meyer's hope for Washington's appreciation.

The *Richmond Times Dispatch* advocated the human conservation plan as a basis for a Virginia state health program. It editorially pointed out that, while the biennial outlay by the state for public health was now $2,222,000, at the same time $17,750,000 were being spent for schools, and $46,000,000 for the roads. ". . . Without minimizing in any way the importance of the schools and the roads, can it reasonably be argued that schools are approximately eight times as important as health, and that roads are about 21 times as important?" asked the *Times Dispatch*. The editorial caught the economics of the human conservation program, ending as follows—

". . . appropriations for health, wisely allotted, can be made to pay tremendous dividends in cash, as well as in a sounder and more stable citizenship."

I V

What mysterious dead hand now lay upon every effort to get the administration and the doctors to stop fighting each other and to begin fighting for the lives and for a now possible higher level of strength of the people? And who was to blame for this misunderstanding? In a notable speech at Jersey City,

New Jersey, on October 2, 1936, the President himself had said—

"Let me with great sincerity give the praise which is due to the doctors and the nurses of the nation for all that they have done during those difficult years that lie behind us, often at great sacrifice, in maintaining the standards of care of the sick and in devoting themselves without reservation to the high ideals of their profession.

"These professions can rest assured that the Federal Administration contemplates no action detrimental to their interests. . . ."

And the American Medical Association, on its side, at the Special Session of its House of Delegates, September, 1938, had held out the olive branch to the federal administration. It had gone on record, in explicit terms, about its determination to co-operate with the government in a health program.

Now what had happened to this beautiful friendship? Now it was May, 1939, at St. Louis, at the annual convention of the American Medical Association, where bitterness and defiance of the government were rampant. The *St. Louis Star-Times*, while anxious to be hospitable to this eminent gathering, registered its distress at certain medical antics in a strong editorial. It began by praising the doctors' atti-

tude toward new ideas in the scientific field. It cele-
brated their genuine devotion to the relief of pain
and suffering. But then—in the matter of their social
viewpoint—this newspaper proceeded to lambaste
them—

"The House of Delegates, the small group of
elected representatives which legislates for the convention, approved a report denouncing the pending
Wagner public health bill in language which sounded
as if it were lifted bodily from the minutes of a meeting of the Liberty League."

The newspaper lamented that the tendency of the
doctors was still one "of inflexibly resisting" any
change in the system by which medical care is
financed almost wholly on an individual physician-
and-patient basis. And who but the most moss-backed
die-hards, who but the stooges of Mr. Frank Gannett, would maintain that the people as individuals
can pay for their care, for their truly adequate treatment, when they're sick? The *Star-Times* did not
thus specifically put the finger on our life-hating die-
hards by name. But it burned the pants off those
medical reactionaries who pretended that this old-
fashioned medical economics worked any longer. "It
is harmful to the people. The majority of families
are unable to afford adequate medical care. Those at

the poverty-income level can obtain attention only on a charity basis. And to the vast middle-income group, a doctor is a luxury not to be contemplated except in dire necessity, when it is often too late."

The indignation of the *St. Louis Star-Times* was high about one "extraordinary" report to the convention, alleging that the number of American people lacking proper medical attention totaled only 40,000. Here the newspaper missed a trick, misreading this remarkable document. It was not in this report maintained that only 40,000 hadn't received proper medical care. It was reported that only 40,000 had been refused it. The *Star-Times* was without intention unjust to the doctors making this report. Surely they deserved praise for their frankness, going on record that the sacred service of relief of pain, healing of sickness, had been refused—

Not to a handful of men, women, and children, but to 40,000 wretched ones. In this rich country.

Of course, what the *Star-Times* writer probably did not know was the off-the-record explanation of this doctor-government bitterness. It wasn't a mere matter of justified medical indignation over crackpot proposals by non-medical framers of the Wagner health bill. The ruckus could not be accounted for on the theory that American medicine is dominated by your gold-digging type of doctor—by those too busy soothing delicate ladies or cutting out genteel appendixes, by those too mercenary to hear the moaning of the poor but proud and in pain, the sobs of the heartbroken, bereaved, because for plain folks good medical care is too expensive. Certain root causes of this brawl—deadly to the people—will probably for a long time remain unpublished. Bitter words had been said, and by high medical luminaries, against the President. On the other hand there had been a tendency in certain government circles to place the medical profession in the well-known zoological group—of so-and-so's. This was more than a split on ideas of how best to lift the level of the health of the people. It had become deeper, more dangerous, because personal—a sub-human feud of medical McCoys and government Hatfields. It seemed that hardly less than squirrel-rifles and sawed-off shotguns could settle this animosity so murderous because so long as it continued there could be no common action to save the lives of the people.

And yet, for all the boisterous hotel-room damnation of Franklin Delano Roosevelt at the St. Louis American Medical Association convention, the ears of certain middle-of-the-road doctors there could detect a theme of whistling in the graveyard in this symphony of defiance. Sensible physicians knew well that this searing editorial in the *St. Louis Star-Times* was no lone voice of the medical woes of America. The powerful and conservative *New York Times*, in brilliant editorials by its sage of science, Mr. Waldemar Kaempffert, reminded the people that all was not well with the care of their sick ones. These sanely progressive A.M.A. doctors knew that the nation needed a better system—economically sound—of bringing together our doctors who alone can give medical care, preventive and curative, and the myriads who need that care but—who dares deny it?—do not now have it.

These liberal physicians—their counsels muffled among recriminations—agreed with the *St. Louis Star-Times* writer when he said that a better health system, stimulated by the government through its Public Health Service, could not long be halted. The people were beginning to know what they wanted. ". . . The people, knowing what they want, will not be frustrated simply because progress can be condemned by an empty catch-phrase such as 'socialized medicine.' "

And the American Medical Association? "If it showed the leadership which might be expected, it would be the most valuable single instrument of progress." On this note ended the *Star-Times* editorial—a sort of Magna Carta it was, for the needlessly sick of the nation.

V

Could these middle-of-the-road liberal doctors be reached, could they learn there was now the possibility of an essentially non-controversial program for human conservation? With the doctors themselves the leaders? With the U. S. Public Health Service technically advising? With the government aiding with a modest amount of money? Was this economic human conservation program, worked upon now for almost five years by our anonymous band of new men against death, sufficiently explicit for the good average public-spirited doctor?

Certain men of medical science to whom the *Country Gentleman's* stories of human erosion and human conservation had been submitted, were heartening in their approval. Microbe hunter Karl F. Meyer, studying them, he said, as he would "a Ph.D. thesis," had only minor criticisms and said the stories were splendid "and just the thing urgently needed." William De Kleine, of the American Red Cross, said they were excellent for the purpose intended, namely to stimulate the legislators. Famed Wisconsin psychiatrist William F. Lorenz felt that "the way the banker was pulled in by the seat of his pants, was good." Lorenz felt the stories would have a tremendous influence and "that our Washington authorities cannot escape a responsibility which is so clearly theirs." Nobel Prizeman George H. Whipple of the University of Rochester—co-conqueror of pernicious anemia—read the manuscripts "with interest and enthusiasm. We can all visualize plenty of difficulties in putting this program into effect, but . . . you are interested in stirring up people to appreciate what can be done and that once done it is an economy rather than a continued expense or a useless expense like armament against imaginary Japanese, Russians, Germans or Italians. . . .

"It is difficult to withhold the use of profanity," wrote Whipple, "when we discuss an attempt to weigh the propriety and usefulness of these two proposals—yours, against those who would crusade to make the world safe against dictators."

Only one among the dozen men of medical science—and he wrote to me wishing himself not quoted—threw cold water on the human conservation program. He called the stories "delightfully vague." He liked no part of government in medicine. This was a blow, because the searcher in question is one of the land's most brilliant students of cancer.

But Michigan's neuro-surgeon Max M. Peet helped to neutralize this criticism by his enthusiasm. "I am in complete agreement on every issue and I believe your suggestion is not a compromise, but a vastly better program than has been suggested by either side. If carried to its possible fruitfulness, much of the social security, group health insurance, etc., would be unnecessary."

Paul O'Leary, famed fighter of syphilis at the Mayo Clinic, and notable for his balance and common sense, said that the stories—

"Gathered together into a workable plan all the sensible schemes and proposals . . . advanced at one time or another in regard to the proposed medical program. I read the stories with the idea of criticizing [them] from the angle of a country doctor and for the life of me I do not see how the A.M.A. crowd can object to the plan. In fact, financially and scientifically your general scheme will put the docs in a better position than they have been before."

Very good. But where to go from here? This was the rub: these were front rank men of medical science, but they were, almost without exception, aloof from the rough-and-tumble of medical politics, national or local, high or low.

Now in June, 1939, came hope, came fire in my guts stoked up by a death fighter not a doctor of medicine. He was Doctor C. C. Young—Cy Young to you—Director of Michigan's State Health Laboratories. He was a microbe hunter, an engineer, a doctor of public health, a servant and immensely respected scientific counselor of Michigan's four-thousand-odd doctors. Young was above and beyond that a servant of Michigan's people. And yet far above and beyond he was the slave of his beautiful state laboratories. With his brain he had built and developed them—for Michigan's physicians, for Michigan's people, sick and healthy. This brain-child of Cy's—and Michigan's best doctors acknowledged it—had been powerful in placing Michigan's physicians in the van of America's death fight.

Cy now brought a strange inspiration to us at Wake Robin where there was, this June—contrary to the loveliness of the woods and the strength of the sun and the life-giving power of Lake Michigan's water—a certain gloom about the possibility of putting a national human conservation program into action. There was this best about Cy Young. He didn't give a damn. He was living on what he called velvet —being one of the few men alive today who had survived, thanks to Hugh Young's surgical genius, an operation for cancer of the kidney. His vast experience in bringing laboratory science into Michigan's practice of medicine made him a man to listen and look up to. His wanting nothing at all for himself, his always giving, giving, made him a man to love and to follow. He looked like a faintly American version of an English colonel. Only brighter.

Now out of his first-hand knowledge he proceeded to state the elements of the problem. There were various kinds of doctors—something that doctor-baiting, health-planning non-medical Washington crackpots did not take into consideration. There are good and bad breeds of cats among doctors, as there are among auto-workers, clergymen, and astrophysicists. There are physicians, said Cy, mainly older ones and not many, who do not want any public check on what they do to, for, or with their patients. According to these surviving die-hards, public health activity should be confined to looking after the water supply, disposing of sewage, supervising handling of public food, furnishing vaccine—free—for smallpox, and tacking up signs for quarantines. Then at the other pole there are certain physicians—mostly young and again few in number—pinko devotees of "red medicine" they've maybe read about in John A. Kingsbury's famed book. They want the state to do everything medical for everybody; they want to try to graft communistic medicine on a capitalistic economic system.

Now caught in the cross-fire between these mossbacks and communizers are the mass of the physicians, not articulate, struggling to practice good medicine and fighting for their livings, not politicians, willing to follow honest physicians whose skill and social wisdom they respect. These are the raw material for the public health army. These are going to have to be the front line fighters for human conservation. And among them—Cy told me he knew them and could put his finger on them—were men dissatisfied with the level of health of the American people, fellows impatient because medical science wasn't now turned on full power.

And here's what we can grab on to, said Cy. There are politically active and powerful doctors among these middle-of-the-road medical progressives. They're not socializers. They're not for the right of every doctor privately and without responsibility to kill or cure patients. They belong to no ism whatever. They do believe—

That health departments should furnish every possible means to every doctor to treat the greatest number of people for prevention and cure of disease —regardless of economic status. Just exactly as cities and states now—nobody objecting—give the best possible equipment to their police, their fire, their conservation departments. They want all scientific and public health aid. But they also want this: to have the responsibility—in their own medical organizations—of the treatment of the sick.

These Michigan doctors are believers in the constitution, and therefore conservatives, said Cy. They believe public health to be a function of government because the constitution of Michigan proclaims that the government of the state of Michigan is responsible for the health and safety of the people of Michigan.

"You don't believe there are such medical animals?" asked Cy with the benign sneer of a veteran immensely more experienced than his pupil. "Well, you should meet a few of them!"

And, said Cy, they existed not only in Michigan, but in every state in the union. They were the white hopes, the without which nothing, of a health program.

VI

Here now in July, 1939, Congress was adjourning without action for a health program. The vast expenditures recommended by the Wagner Health Bill were—so the grapevine had it—out of the question with the national administration. The Wagner Health Bill hearings had dissolved into the futility so characteristic of democratic statesmanship, or rather the lack of it. Washington high command was having a wonderful time, playing on the floor with battleships, tanks, soldiers and fourteen thousand new bombing and fighting planes—think of it. Possible action for human life was unthinkable by those preoccupied with getting ready for America's share in the coming *danse macabre*.

Was there any hope of organizing a pressure group? To tell the country? To tell the national administration that it would be a long time before we'd need all these deadly toys? And that, meanwhile, people were needlessly sick and dying? And that, anyway, it wouldn't be a bad idea to begin right now with a health program that would give our great warriors a more fit America to man those battleships, tanks, and airplanes? A meeting was called in July in

Philadelphia to discuss the possibility of organizing such a pressure group—a people's lobby for public health.

Editor Philip S. Rose presided. There was something pathetic about our entirely informal gathering of volunteer laymen against death. We had no—*standing's* the word for it. We were only a bunch of plain citizens feeling round for a way to crystallize the will of the people for human conservation. There was not one physician here. Doc O'Connor—who was there—thought it might be possible to interest some of the eminent Americans who were trustees of the National Foundation for Infantile Paralysis. But they were very, very busy men, very, very big shots. David M. Noyes—having come here with eight broken ribs, hardly able to move, after an auto accident—believed he might interest Mr. A. D. Lasker. That *might* bring in the powerful publicity machinery of the Lord and Thomas advertising agency. Yet we did not know where to begin.

Philip Rose had made a clear statement of the *Country Gentleman's* platform for the health of the American people. It had been published in the form of the stories on human erosion and human conservation. Walter Fuller, Fred Healy, and Cary Bok of the Curtis Publishing Company said they were back of Phil Rose's proposals. There was no strife, and the hearts of the little meeting beat as one and the minds had but a single thought. But how to go about really organizing a people's lobby? We lacked confidence. We lacked some basic element—without which our plans and hopes were moonshine.

Now Cy Young told us what it really was that we were wanting and had not got. Miserably paid public servant of Michigan that he was, Cy had flown to this meeting at his own expense. Now he electrified us. For thirty minutes he gave us, not beautiful dreams of a public health utopia, but the lowdown. Here's what had to be done before we could even begin to ask the people to roar their demand for public health—

We had to have the organized medical profession back of the human conservation idea.

We had to tell the doctors—and the American people—*that public health is good for doctors.*

We had to tell the doctors and the American people *that public health needs the doctors.* Cy did not talk generalities. He gave hard facts, cold figures. He overwhelmed us. Then when the doctors became one with the people—when at last they took their proper place of leading the people in the demand for public health—then would be the time to try to organize the mass lobby for human conservation. That was the way to get action.

Phil Rose said okay. He said to go ahead and write those stories. The *Country Gentleman* would publish them. This, then, that follows is Cy Young's plan, distilled out of his immense practical experience, with the doctors, with the people. So I went back to Wake Robin to write these stories. In an expanded form in the following three chapters they are here presented, substantially as printed in the *Country Gentleman*.

V. Public Health Is Good for Doctors *

IT IS not strange that there has been antagonism between the ancient profession of medicine and the upstart profession of public health. It is remarkable that, in their common fight against death, our doctors and healthmen pull together as well as they do. Because, in the line of his duty, the public healthman has had to step onto the most sacred ground, into the intimate relation between patient and doctor. In the old days, before medical science gave doctors power actually to save life, they were accountable only to themselves for the life or death of their individual patients. It was a terrific prerogative. If you were gravely sick, and lived, it was the doctor who pulled you through. If you died, it was not the doctor who had killed you. It was an act of God. Engineers might be discredited if their bridges collapsed under railroad trains, with loss of life. Generals were deposed when their bungling led to butchery of armies. Political leaders, held responsible for the people's

* Substantially as printed in *Country Gentleman*, October 1939.

133

misery and hunger, were beheaded or voted out of power. But your doctor? This was his special privilege: that your death was his own damn business.

Then came science, came the beginnings of the actual power, not the mere amiable pretense of physicians to save our lives. Then too came bookkeepers of life and death—these were the health officers. Was this particular death curable, preventable? The public healthmen published the death rates for all citizens to know. They turned the terrible searchlight of their figures on life and death onto that old sacred ground—doctor: patient—where none had walked before. So, for the first time in history, our doctors were put upon the spot in the matter of life and death. The new medical science gave them the new power—miraculous—of actually saving human life. Now the healthmen asked a new discipline of the doctors: to give an accounting of those who died. So it is not to be wondered at that certain physicians fret under this transformation of their old mysterious medical art into public science. Some old-fashioned doctors even feel public healthmen to be their natural enemies, accuse them of plots to socialize medicine, to take the care of the sick away from the physicians.

On the other hand, as our fantastically expanding power of medical science makes it possible to con-

quer more and more death, the co-fighting against
death of the best physicians and public healthmen
has become all the time closer. Now, if we are to be
honestly able to assure our political leaders that we
are today ready to launch a national health program,
this doctor-public healthman co-operation must become complete, unquestioning.

That's entirely possible, when public healthmen
once realize how they're nothing without the physicians; and when doctors see clearly how good public
health has already been for them, how it can add to
the power and the glory of their fight against death.

I I

It is true that, compared to the ancient profession
of medicine, the origin of healthmen is recent. Their
beginnings were humble. Before the coming of medical science the one duty of health officers—Paul
Revere was the first one in America—was "to remove all filth of any kind whatever . . . whenever
such filth shall in their judgment endanger the lives
or health of the inhabitants."

What kept the health officers at the level of mere
scavengers was this: that there was no science to tell
them whether the dirt they were removing was

merely a nuisance—or deadly. But even so, in those pre-scientific days of the 19th century, the doctors should not have looked down their noses too much at health officers. Because for the doctors there was no science, either, to tell them whether they were curing or killing their patients!

Then arose the microbe hunters, the new men against death, bringing death-fighting truth. This revolutionized—and simultaneously—the twin professions of medicine and public health. And this new basic science put the ancient physicians and the upstart healthmen—willy-nilly—into one and the same death-fighting army. Your physician had still to soothe the brows of individual typhoid fever patients at bedsides, but it was no longer a private sickness to be fought solely by bedside doctors. Microbe hunters—not privileged often to write "M.D." after their names—traced the sneakings of the typhoid microbe. Engineers—sometimes with no learned letters after their names at all—disposed of the sewage, purified the water, pasteurized the milk that carried typhoid death from one human being to the next one. Where doctors saved one life, these new non-medical men saved thousands. . . .

The power of this new sanitary science was so terrific that, between 1911 and 1935, the typhoid death rate tumbled twentyfold in our country. It was inevitable that our physicians became involved in a new kind of public bookkeeping, an accounting for mass saving of human life. . . . Their intimate struggle for one life in one sickroom became submerged in the promise that this new science could wipe out the curse of typhoid fever—forever.

Now our healthmen began to perform other services for the doctors. They became links between laboratory science and the practicing physicians. Health departments—from their laboratories—began giving family doctors free death-fighting ammunition. First, serum to cure many cases of diphtheria. Then toxoid, to prevent, to wipe out that sickness. The doctors themselves were the proud front line soldiers, using these miraculous weapons. The healthman's vital statistics showed the doctors their victory; eight times fewer children died this choking death in 1935 than in 1911.

Consumption was a personal secret between the bedside doctor and its victim till the turn of the century. Then healthmen stepped in, requiring that all cases of this death be reported, recorded. In 1911, it was head killer of Americans. It would surely have remained so if microbe hunters, x-ray experts, healthmen, nurses, chest-surgeons hadn't begun co-working with the family physicians, finding all cases, isolating them, curing them—fighting it as mass, not individual, death. Fighting not TB but the TB death rate. By 1935 this new death-fighting team had dragged TB down to seventh place among killers.

In eight American cities in 1900 the death of babies the first year they were born was at the ghastly total of four hundred out of every thousand born alive. The wisest physicians, alone at cradlesides, admitted they could not stem this mass slaughter of innocents. They could only comfort parents, saying it still was—well—the old alibi, the will of God. Again, non-medical allies came to help the physicians. Free milk stations for poor families began to develop into child health centers. Here the doctors and public health nurses began teaching mothers how to feed strength into their youngsters, began teaching them hygiene. Healthmen directed the pasteurizing of death out of milk.

Down, too, now went infant death, all over.

Down to an all time low, in Chicago, 1936, only thirty-eight babies dying of every thousand born alive. Instead of four hundred per thousand!

Public healthmen began to drag their nets for lurking sickness and death through public schools, reporting their discoveries to family doctors. This was the difference between the old bedside medicine and the new applied medical science: keeping tab on sickness and death rates made you—willy-nilly— think of sickness and death, made you fight them, in mass. And what happened at bedsides, important, was only one link in the chain of the new fight for life. Each death rate lowered was thanks not only to physicians. These were now part of a new kind of health army—not regimented, but voluntary, with engineers, microbe hunters, doctors, chemists, nurses, pathologists, public healthmen, all soldiers. And all indispensable.

In the first third of this present century the individual conquests of death rates, like those above recorded, began to total up into a momentous general decrease in America's rate of dying. In this death fight there was a democracy, an attempt—though far from perfect—to give equal chance for life to all people, regardless. Doctor Louis I. Dublin has charted the up of the life, the down of the death, of seventeen million industrial policy holders of a great insurance company. They're a cross section of Americans, workers and their families. From 1911 to 1935, Dublin has calculated and condensed their dying into one simple line. It has a majestic sweep, down and down. That line is the most simple diagram of mankind's new power over nature. The dislocations of the first world war did nothing to stem that death line's down trend. During all those twenty-five years there was just one short interruption, from the flu, the most deadly epidemic in the memory of living man. Even the worst economic tailspin in our country's history did nothing to halt the improved chances of living, of Dublin's seventeen million average Americans. Thanks to the doctors. Thanks to the healthmen.

III

Even so, who dares to say that this new health army headed by healthmen and doctors is alone responsible for this mass triumph over death? There remain mysteries about our present amazing low general death rate of less than nine per thousand population. Part credit must go, maybe, to human activities in which death fighting was not the intention. Strange forces have been at work—influences not human at all.

The four horsemen of death of children—diphtheria, scarlet fever, measles, whooping cough—all faded in their killing power from 1911 to 1935. Yet only against diphtheria did our men of medical science have a preventive and a cure. What force weakened the savagery of the microbes of whooping cough and scarlet fever? What made the virus of measles less deadly? How sure are we that our boasted weapons—even against tuberculosis—have been alone, or principally, responsible for the white death's slow fading?

That is the beauty of their science; that is the impersonal power of our public healthmen. Their bookkeeping does not try to justify their jobs, their existence. Their bookkeeping is science, cold, analytical, asking embarrassing self-questions—the remote opposite of the ancient belief that when you got well, it was doc who'd cured you, and when you died, it was an act of God. Here was honesty, refusing to take credit for life-saving that had happened in spite of you. And here was the chance to search for some unsuspected death fighting force.

Was it, maybe, that vague, not precisely measurable thing called the rising American standard of living that had fought scarlet fever, measles, whooping cough? From magazines, radio, movies, newspapers, people have learned about healthfuller houses. From this propaganda American mothers have got a science—crude but powerful—of feeding health into their children. Then too automobiles have taken families out into life-giving fresh air and sun. Families have become smaller, so crowding in houses grows less. Was it then this rising standard of life that toughened our children? It seemed so—when healthmen could record how these mortalities still bore heavily upon the youngsters of the very poor.

But even among these, scarlet fever has not the deadly virulence of old. Must we be too proud of our death-fighting prowess? Is it partly coincidence —that as our science develops, the old deaths happen to be waning? Probing into the living and dying of his seventeen millions, Doctor Dublin has found something other than the rising American standard of living that came to the aid of our men against death. An absolutely not human force, a terrible human disaster, helped to drive that death line down. This ally of our health army was death itself! The line of our dying had been going gradually down-hill from 1911 through 1917. Then the flu pandemic exploded. It killed more than ten million people the world over, 1918-19. In our country the mass flu murder for the first time interrupted the down-trending death line, sent it sharply upward, but for a few months only. And then, fantastic—

With the burning out of the great epidemic, the curve went down. Not down to where it had been before. But something jolted it down to a much lower level. And it kept on going downward from that lower figure. Now, instead of thirteen per one thousand people dying as they had been dying before the flu, 1917, in 1921 that figure had dropped to nine per thousand!

It cannot be accounted for on the explanation that the flu cleaned out a lot of weaklings who in the next few years would anyway have died. The flu cleaned out the young and strong. . . .

Did the flu, infecting more than half our population, destroy some other lurking, but completely unknown, death in the vast majority who after all did not die from flu, but were simply sick with it? Did flu make them—some way—healthier people? Or among the hundreds of thousands who did die from the flu, was some still mysterious infection of another kind buried underground with them? So it could not attack our surviving people in the years thereafter?

This shows again how public health is good for doctors. It makes them less cocksure of the power of the science they have now. Our true medical leaders do not squabble with public healthmen over who has done how much to send our general death rate downward. Both of them know it was a little half-paralyzed man with neither an M.D. or a D.P.H.

after his name—Louis Pasteur—who is to be thanked
for this greatest of all steps forward in human history. And the best doctors and public healthmen are
brothers in humility before the veil still shrouding
the unknown reasons why we live or die. They know
the still feeble power of their best science. And they
are honest—

They are honest with the people. They are not
smug about the alleged high level of health in our
country where the rate of dying has sunk so relatively low. They do not stop to congratulate themselves—unctuously cutting the medical and public
health professions large pieces of cake—because
America's general death rate is lower than that of
any country in the world. They do not pull the wool
over the eyes of our citizens, crying out and pointing,
"Lo here! Lo there!" to the plague in India, the
malaria in Brazil, the typhus in Russia, the dysentery
in China.

These foreign disasters do not blind our public-
spirited doctors and healthmen to our own terrible
public health problems, our own needless human
erosion.

And here again public healthmen are ready to
suggest new battles to doctors now maybe despairing
that we have become so healthy that there will soon

be little left for the physicians to do! The health-men, by their vital statistics, have mapped out and plotted new fields to conquer. They are ready to take jaded physicians, sighing for more sickness and death to conquer—

Into insane asylums to live among gibbering, vacant-eyed wretches. Into slums to spend a few weeks with myriads rotting to death with tuberculosis because institutions do not exist for their care and cure. Into hospital wards to spend days and nights at bedsides of forlorn ones wanting only death's mercy to end their torture from cancer. Into dingy workers' hovels, to comfort mothers wondering how they are going to feed their already undernourished children, now that the breadwinner has been killed by pneumonia. Into shacks reeking with the ammoniacal aroma of poverty—to learn why children, born healthy, are wrecked by rheumatic heartbreak. Into houses, in farm and city, of rich as well as poor, to condole with mothers over crippled, spastic children and to comfort children uncared for by invalid mothers—all the aftermath of bungling care of mothers at childbirth. They can visit, too, homes where breadwinners are jobless because of rheumatism, or laid off from work because of failing hearts. Then there are hundreds of thousands of families to see, where the pale spirochete of syphilis is guest, where little children are very gentle, not mischievous, and have bulging foreheads, and where other children are slowly going blind, or where a once happy family is wrecked. . . . By the loss of the job of a once competent father . . . who at last lapses into homicidal madness.

I V

Old-fashioned doctors are still to be found who believe that public health takes the bread out of honest physicians' mouths. The opposite is true. In states like New York, Massachusetts, Michigan and others where public health activity is highly developed, it puts a formidable amount of money into the pockets of practicing doctors. Doctor C. C. Young has estimated the portion of the average physician's earnings resulting directly from public health activities in Michigan.

This is Doctor Young's calculation of the cash value of what public health does, yearly, for the state's practicing physicians and their organizations—

Food handlers in Michigan are required to undergo medical examination, to prevent them from carrying disease. The doctor is selected by the individual to be examined. Seventy-five thousand of these examinations are made. Fee: not less than one dollar per examination. For doctors—$75,000.

Over 350,000 school children are sent to doctors for first office calls for the correction of some defect or other, detected while they're at school. Minimum charge, a dollar for each call. For physicians— $350,000.

—Nobody knows how many subsequent office calls follow from these first visits—

Each year, the Health Department Laboratories, testing blood of citizens for syphilis, find more than seven thousand new cases of this disease. One hundred dollars a case is a low estimate of the doctor's charge. For the practitioner—$700,000. This does not include cases found at pre-marital examinations.

The State Health Department Laboratories distribute vaccines, tuberculin, and other disease-preventing and disease-diagnosing products, free in Michigan. But somebody has to give them, namely, the practicing doctor. Two hundred thousand doses of these products are yearly distributed. A charge of one dollar per inoculation is conservative. For the physicians—$200,000.

—This does not include smallpox vaccine, also distributed free, because, says Doctor Young, much smallpox vaccination is done for nothing. Yet recently, in a Michigan city, smallpox broke out among performers in a circus. The State Health Department acted promptly, vaccinating two hundred circus employees to scotch the epidemic. This public action led directly to doctors privately vaccinating more than three thousand people of the community—

Before marrying, Michigan's men and women must undergo examination for venereal disease. Last year this caused doctors to uncover over one thousand hitherto unsuspected cases of syphilis. For the pre-marital examinations $200,000 is a conservative estimate of money going to Michigan's physicians. For treating the new cases—a minimum of $100,000.

Michigan law makes provision for medical and hospital care for crippled and afflicted children. Last year the charge upon the state for this public service by doctors and hospitals was $2,900,000.

Rabies vaccine for people bitten by mad dogs and lockjaw antitoxin are manufactured and distributed free by the state laboratories to Michigan's doctors. Last year 60,000 doses of rabies vaccine and 50,000 doses of lockjaw serum were sent to practitioners for their private use on patients. Low estimate of income to doctors for these inoculations—$110,000.

Doctor Young concludes that Michigan's public

health activity of various kinds means annual cash income of $4,635,000 for doctors and their organizations.

There are four thousand physicians in the state. The average income of doctors in America is said to be about $3,000. That would put the total income of Michigan's doctors at a figure of the order of $12,000,000. So the contribution made by public health to the doctor is a formidable one.

And public health is good not only for the doctors of the state of Michigan. A similar estimate of what public health does for New York State's doctors was made under direction of New York State Health Commissioner Edward S. Godfrey, Jr. The income—thanks to public health activity—for upstate New York's doctors approximates closely that of Michigan's physicians.

V

Some die-hard doctors may still insist that in spite of this, health departments and health officers are really making havoc of the old relationship, patient-doctor. Again, in Michigan, Cy Young shows how the exact opposite is true. The state's healthmen do everything they can to lead the people to the practicing physician. The last thing the healthmen want to do is to undertake the care of the sick. They know they're not capable of it. They believe it must remain the doctors' responsibility.

At the same time it is perfectly clear that there's no longer a sharp line between preventive and curative medicine. But this is what public healthmen believe they must do: namely, furnish all doctors every technical weapon they need and do not have for the prevention and cure of the sickness of all the people. Cy Young's superb Michigan State Health Department Laboratories are a model for this public health aid to the state's practicing physicians. The laboratories furnish free to the state's doctors all the most effective and generally used vaccines, serums, toxoids. They demonstrate to the doctors anything they may need to know about their proper use. They remove from the physician the financial burden he used to have, of carrying accounts of these products on his own private books.

But the actual use of these weapons? That is between the physician and his individual patient.

Michigan's laboratories further perform—and again it is a free service—all tests the state's doctors may have to have made to uncover communicable diseases. They make other tests, highly technical, for diseases not contagious, where the patient is unable to pay for private laboratory services.

Do the doctors use this public health service? They themselves answer—by the fact that the state laboratories now make over six hundred thousand of such examinations, yearly, for practicing physicians. Does this take bread out of the mouths of the doctors? The doctors themselves answer: as a result of information given them by these laboratory examinations, thousands of patients begin treatment for diabetes, pernicious anemia, venereal and other diseases. At the hands of Michigan's private practitioners.

Not only its state laboratories, but in general Michigan's public health services, guide the people to the doctors. Public healthmen and public health nurses teach women to consult their physicians before they marry, and to go to doctors for prenatal care, the moment they know they are going to have babies—

All school boards are requested to require a physical and x-ray examination of teachers entering their profession, and every two years thereafter. This work is done by the physician of the teacher's own choice—

Many industries in Michigan require a doctor's certificate to the effect that the applicant for a job is free from occupational disease. The examination is paid for by the worker. To the doctor he himself chooses.

Public health officers of cities, counties, and the state, keep up widespread, incessant, teaching and preaching to every sort of group of Michigan's people—to businessmen's clubs, churches, P.T.A.'s, women's clubs, granges, lodges, schools. They are told that health is purchasable. They are told to go to their doctors to buy it.

The business thus sent into doctors' offices is not directly calculable. Any honest doctor will admit it is formidable and that it adds greatly to the more than $4,000,000 above mentioned.

Finally, Michigan's state health department is developing a service to keep such practicing physicians —as may want to—abreast of the advances in medical science, in the care of mothers in childbirth, in the uncovering and treatment of syphilis, in the early diagnosis of cancer. So that the practicing physicians may better meet the needs of the thousands of people sent them—by public health.

Even so, in their organization of a volunteer health army of public healthmen and physicians, Michigan's men know that only a beginning has been made of a now possible battle against disease now preventable, or curable if it is found early.

And this is true of the volunteer health armies of New York, Massachusetts, and every state in the union. All need more laboratory services. All need more and better-distributed laboratories and health centers. All need training for doctors in our marvelously developing science. All need money to help the doctors bring this life-saving science to the masses of the people who have not got the money to pay for the health and life that science can give them.

Michigan's public-spirited doctors know that localities, counties, the state itself, are not financially able to furnish all the money needed for the powerful weapons demanded by a modern health army. Far better than our national administration, Michigan's physicians seem to appreciate it that, for health, the horse-and-buggy days are over. They know that the microbes, the diseases, and, yes, the people hit by sickness have no regard for state boundaries in our automobile nation, our highly migratory America. Michigan's doctors would like to run their own health program, would like to show the country how they can organize to take care of their own sick folks—

They are getting ready to show America that the doctors of this state now consider health—and the best-known care of it—to be the fifth human right.

But they would certainly welcome technical advice and help from Washington.

And they know there must be a national health program—co-ordinated and federally advised—and aided according to local needs by federal money.

It is stirring to see these physicians becoming—healthmen. When national medico-political leaders tell Michigan's doctors that our health progress has been wonderful, those doctors say, yes, that's right, but in their own communities the still terrible ravages of sickness and death are before their eyes. They know that no sickness and death rate is a good rate till it's as low as their medical science can make it. They are not wasteful; in the enormous majority they are not chiselers and grafters.

They wonder why the national administration is so strongly opposed to expanding present feeble federal grants in aid of their now possible fight for the lives of Michigan's people.

VI. Public Health Needs the Doctors *

THE MYSTIC might of science tends to transform the old-fashioned physician into a new breed of man. He seems significant beyond any men in human history. Such is the truly modern doctor. He is not afraid to be called a death fighter. He is highly conscious of this duty, yet not arrogant because of it. Fulfilling it, he is incorruptible. It is granted that, among our nation's one hundred and fifty thousand physicians, there are not yet many thus completely dedicated. Still, so great and more and more pervading is the power of science that there remain today few physicians who have not savored the experience of man's new dominion over death. Till now —though this must change!—our healers are not deliberately chosen from better human stuff than ordinary. Yet the plainest doctor today, looking down at a desperately sick man or woman, can now and again answer—NO!—

* Substantially as printed in *Country Gentleman*, December 1939.

155

When that human being begs him: "Doctor, you won't let me die?"

More and more the physician dares to make this answer, not fooling. Not pretending, because, as in pre-scientific days, death would come to cover up the falseness of that promise. Now he promises life to the doomed one. More and more the promise is redeemed. Yes, the physician fails, and often. He bungles, unskilled to use the new weapons, subtle as they are powerful. His fumbling hands may kill. It is his awful discipline and secret tragedy to learn by the very death of those who might have been kept alive by hands more deft, by judgment surer. Yet, more and more the average doctor—though not a dedicated death fighter—tastes this new salt of life—

The rescue of a man, or woman, or child who if stricken ten years, five years, one year, yes, one week earlier, must needs have died . . .

This giving of a lease on life where death had heretofore been fore-ordained smacks of the miraculous, though it stems from plain facts and reason. We can forgive our physician for the residue of quack-salving humbug clinging to medical practice because of this new and godlike power. For this we value him above all other human beings. For all his pretentious clothing of simple scientific fact in Latin jargon, we realize that now and again, and more and more, he shoots magic bullets against our death, with clear eye and hands that do not tremble.

The rank and file of physicians today are not yet easy in this new post of honor. Because they now show us flashes of this new and seeming supernatural power, they bear a terrible responsibility, and not toward individual patients only. The doctors sense this—and why should it not irk them?—that we begin to hold them accountable for the lives of all. It isn't this one child cured of yesterday's surely deadly streptococcus meningitis; or this one mother moribund with pneumonia but now living; or this one father, doomed with cancer, and saved to earn his children's bread; or this wee boy, once lame, now walking. These miracles and dozens as marvelous are daily front page stories and astound us. But they are not enough.

There is a human intuition—call it religious—that makes the ultimate distribution of this new mercy to all inevitable. This is the human belief—silly to the snobbish—that the saving of one human being makes the needless dying of all other infamous. So mankind asks, not whispering it but making it peremptory, official:

How many remain miserable, bereft of reason,

racked and crippled from ills preventable and curable? And why, doctor, do you let any of these die?

This is public health. Thus is the ancient chicanery of the laying on of hands, the physicking, being transformed into the modern science of medicine. And the physician emerges from his ancient priestcraft, as each human being that he saves becomes not only an object of affection but also a statistic, another unit to be subtracted from the death rate. His role is immensely more difficult than that of the healthman for whom human beings are statistics only.

Here is a fact not longer to be evaded by our doctors: they, the practitioners, are the spearhead of this human advance now beginning to gain momentum.

They first see sufferers at bedsides.

Intimate with sickness and health of their families in their practices, doctors only can spot illness in its first stages, can head off death before it threatens.

They are the shock troops against the nation's needless dying. No national health program can even be thought of without them. Public health more than needs our doctors. It demands them.

II

But this must be faced: that there are still many physicians who resist public health expansion. There are not a few for whom medicine remains—business. There exists among some the fantastic fear that prevention of disease—as science turned on full power could now prevent it—will abolish the doctor's reason for being. This was not long ago actually expressed by an old-fashioned Michigan doctor who told it to that modern Michigan doctor, L. G. Christian. The old doctor's boy wanted to follow in his father's footsteps. "Don't think of it, my son," admonished the old healer. "You won't make a living. Diphtheria's going. Pretty soon there won't be any TB. Why, *my* father put me through school on typhoid fever!"

Yet it is a fact that for every death near conquered, there is another malady, the prevention and cure of which gives wide-awake physicians the chance to be busier than ever. And this is the essence of the one sound national health program: it will stir our doctors, of their own free will, to become public healthmen in their private practices. The beginnings of such a program are to be seen in more than one state, and notably in New York State, where doctors and public healthmen have joined to fight death—instead of each other.

Acting as volunteer healthmen in the war on syphilis, upstate New York's physicians are giving hundreds of thousands of treatments to make a start of wiping out this plague.

The New York State Medical Society has agreed with the State Health Department to co-operate in an attempt to cut down the pneumonia death rate—with serum, and now with the magic chemical sulfapyridine.

Aided by the state's laboratories and health department, New York's doctors last year spotted thousands of new cases of cancer, many in time for cure.

In a dozen other death fights the state's rank and file doctors are getting the healthman's slant: examining children in schools, detecting early TB, caring for crippled children, giving serums and vaccines provided free—as in Michigan—by the state's laboratories. . . .

Yet the best of the state's doctors are not smug about New York's death rate in 1938 being lower than ever in its history. The best ones raise their eyes, look beyond the bedside of this one sick human being—over to the death rate curves calculated by their state health department. These are the challenge. These accuse them of the still needless dying of thousands, of the life-wreck of countless others. New York's public-health-minded doctors do not stop to celebrate the down-trending death lines for children under five, youngsters under fourteen, young grownups under twenty-four. After all, the death curve of grownups from twenty-five to forty-four has not gone so brilliantly. The death rates of men and women in prime of life—forty-five to sixty-four—trends ominously upward. That is the new battleground in the death fight upstate New York is organizing. The state health department has broken down the causes of the death of the people. Three out of four deaths are caused by ten diseases—led by the three master killers: heart disease, cancer, and pneumonia.

The fight cannot be purely medical. All but three of these ten chief killing sicknesses have been proved to have a formidable ally. Against it the skill and science of the practicing physician avails nothing. The ally of these seven deaths is poverty. This friend of death would ruin doctors, too, if they fought these deaths on the old basis of every man paying his own doctor. Public co-operation—in a manner acceptable to physicians—is demanded.

III

Third highest among these ten killers, powerfully aided by poverty, stands pneumonia. Upstate New York, it kills more than three thousand people yearly. It bears most heavily upon poor people. At the same time—as of 1937—its cure is a costly business. What then could the private physician do but let such people die?

In addition to its unfair preference for the poor folks, pneumonia plays another vicious trick upon humanity and the doctors. It's far the easiest to cure in the very first hours of the sickness when the victim, hoping to get by with just a bad chest cold, does not call his physician. At the same time it is notorious that private physicians do not go into homes, even of families they know most intimately, to find sickness. It is unethical. So how could New York's doctors get at those sick ones who do not realize that from this "bad chest cold," in four or five days they may be dead?

It has been medically published that the Medical Society of the State of New York asked the help of the State Health Department in this dilemma. The low-down has it that, as far back as 1935, the State

Health Department went down on its knees—figuratively—to ask the practicing doctors to use the new serum—free. That doesn't matter. What is important is that the doctors and the state's healthmen now both enjoy the credit of pioneering in the state's present hopeful fight against pneumonia.

The first step was economic. The State Legislature was convinced that it is far more costly for a community to maintain pneumonia deaths than to prevent them. The unheard-of sum of $400,000 was appropriated for pneumonia serum—free, for any doctor who's trained to use it.

The first serum was powerful only against the widely prevalent, highly murderous Type I pneumonia. But since any one of thirty other types of pneumonia microbes might hit New York's citizens, the health department, through a statewide chain of approved laboratories, saw to it that quick testing for type of pneumonia was at hand—free—for the upstate doctors.

—Curiously there was no howl about this step into what moss-backs might call "state medicine"—

Now the serum treatment of pneumonia is a highly technical business, and where were the specialists to defend sufferers from this death, especially out in the country? It is an interesting fact that the most implacable saboteurs of a national health program are certain medical political leaders who lament that physicians are not technically equipped to use the new science. Among certain medical bigwigs there is obvious contempt for the medical rank and file. Now, acting as the agent of the State Medical Society, health department experts organized institutes, group conferences. They rapidly and successfully turned upstate New York's town and country physicians into pneumonia specialists.

Yet what good this medical skill, this free serum, if the ordinary citizen does not understand the desperate need to call a doctor before pneumonia's got him desperately sick? Here New York's public health and medical death fighters were confronted by another bogey—it is frequently erected by anti-health program medical politicoes—the fear that your average citizen is too ignorant to even want the science now ready to save him! This dirty libel of the average American did not daunt New York's doctors. They threw overboard the fusty ethics that required them to wait—dignified in their offices—for people in peril to call them. They went out to scotch the pneumonia killer before he'd become too formidable. The town and country doctors now made talks—prepared for them by State Health Department experts

—to community meetings, organized by Farm and Home Bureaus.

They stripped the medical bedside mystery of its mumbo jumbo. They taught plain citizens to begin to diagnose their own pneumonia! They told people to call their doctors, when they first felt bad, head-achy, chilly, feverish, and suffered that first stab of chest pain—

That winter nearly nine hundred formerly rank and file physicians practiced this specialty of pneu-monia cure upon thousands of pneumonia sufferers. Over five hundred of these were treated in farm homes, not hospitals. Death from pneumonia Type I —very common—was far below that dreadful one-in-three who die when not given serum the first few days of their sickness.

Could the doctors learn to be effective teachers of the people—when from time's beginning it had been medical ethics to keep medicine mysterious to laymen? In the grave pneumonia epidemic in rural Wyoming County in western New York—1938 Winter—seventy out of every hundred sufferers were under treatment in that county's excellent hos-pital within forty-eight hours of the beginning of their danger.

Already upstate New York's doctors, less and less

secretly proud to be public healthmen, have saved hundreds of people who would otherwise surely have perished. The state pneumonia death rate is on the down-grade. But now comes news of the new chemical miracle—sulfapyridine—acting against all types of pneumonia, regardless. And twenty times cheaper than the powerful serum! And so mighty against pneumococcus microbes that—so says famed expert Perrin H. Long of the Johns Hopkins Hospital—next to nobody, adequately treated with sulfapyridine on the first day of pneumonia—will die.

Good news, yes, but there's still better for hundreds of thousands of Americans yearly faced by this third greatest of all death's dangers. The best news of all is the way this public health spirit of New York's doctors is spreading through the medical rank and file. It is shown by an outburst, made last summer by Michigan's Doctor L. G. Christian. Greg Christian is a delegate to the national organization of doctors, to the American Medical Association. He is one of that great guild's governing body. He is highly on to the ropes of medical politics and loves it. Is the practice of medicine still the private right of the doctor to cure his patient or to let him die? Not for Greg Christian.

"With serum and especially this new drug," says

Greg, his eyes beaming behind his spectacles, "if we could just catch all the state's pneumonia in the first twenty-four hours, we'd knock the death rate down to next to nothing! Like we've already done with diphtheria. By God, we'll do it!"

This is the writing on the wall for those who are still of the belief that the people will be best served by keeping medicine a private matter. We know that Christian's is more than a lone, a free-lance voice in medicine.

I V

When your patient's life and death is your own damn business, you, the doctor, do not have to be open; there are times when it is best for you not to be honest. It is notorious that medical self-criticism, if it existed in the now happily dying quack-salving days, was not heard by the people. Now this changes, as doctors join with the public healthmen to fight the death of all. 1937, the Medical Society of Ingham County, Michigan, began a truly historical fight against syphilis. It is the first public survey of physicians by those physicians themselves, they telling their failures and faults ahead of their virtues.

With some timidity in the autumn of 1937, public-spirited urologist, Bob Breakey, of Lansing, Michigan, suggested to Greg Christian that the Ingham County doctors wanted to consult with Surgeon General Parran of the U. S. Public Health Service. The physicians knew syphilis to be rampant in their county. They wanted Parran's advice and help. But—

"Go on, put it up to him," urged Christian. "What's scaring you? Who the hell is Parran? He's just the Surgeon General, that's all. He's working for you, isn't he?"

So Breakey and his colleagues waited upon the courteous, gray-haired Surgeon General—that "little man" at Washington. They reported to Parran that ninety-seven per cent of the doctors of their county had voted as willing to draw blood for the syphilis test—from every single patient in their practices. Regardless of what might apparently be ailing them . . .

It was a bold plan. It was risky for every doctor. God knows, these hard times, they need every paying patient. And what if their prize patients should be insulted by their good doctor's so much as suspecting they'd ever been within a mile of a syphilis spirochete? Now Parran—that night at Wake Robin telling how stirred and touched he's been by this plea from this little delegation of embryo public healthmen—proceeded to put the facilities of the U. S. Public Health Service at the Ingham County Medical Society's disposal. Now from mid-January to mid-March, 1938, guided by Public Health Service experts, these Michigan volunteer healthmen, practicing doctors all, worked their blood-test dragnet through their patients of high and low degree.

—Another bogey exploded. There is no record of any patient being insulted by proposal of a blood test—

Now the doctors did an Emile Zola on themselves. Here was the state of the health of Ingham County, Michigan, in regard to syphilis, in regard to which these doctors now proceeded to accuse themselves—

Five out of six of the cases found by their blood tests had never been treated for syphilis.

Syphilis is a legally reportable disease in Michigan. But there were forty per cent more cases under treatment by the county's practicing physicians than had been reported to the health authorities.

The doctors could not hold their patients under treatment! Only one out of every three cases of syphilis was being treated long enough to make the sufferer not dangerous to other people of the community.

Just as the doctors were falling down as public healthmen, so they were falling down as—physicians. Because five out of six people were not being treated thoroughly enough to be surely guarded against the final disasters of syphilitic heart-wreck or of insanity.

Here were doctors who dared to become economists, who dared to be honest about everything *not* being all right in this best of all possible worlds of American medical practice. For every patient who could afford to pay the physician for the admittedly expensive treatment of syphilis—there were nine too poor to do so.

When people who ran out of money, for this reason lapsed their treatment, the doctors were not generally reporting such lapses to the health authorities. Though all these victims were running at large, and many were dangerous to the community.

The Ingham County doctors were failing as syphilis detectives. They were finding a lot of syphilis. They were treating it. They were failing to find out from whom their patients had caught the plague or to whom they might be giving it.

Such was their self-searching. It came from no public scandal about their incompetence. Those doctors investigated their public health incompetence, but, far more important, they aired it. As a medical organization, among all county medical societies in the nation, they made history—

They went on record as acknowledging that the practicing physician should hold himself accountable for all syphilis existing in his community.

Then they went further. It cannot have been a nice pill for the let-us-alones high in organized medicine's councils. They admitted that they, the practitioners, could not wipe this shame from Ingham County. If not aided by public healthmen. Here's the public help they needed—

They must have an epidemic expert to work out of their offices, to track down where every case of syphilis comes from, and to follow people to whom syphilis will try to go. Government help was asked to hire this syphilis detective. They wanted to try to treat all discoverable syphilis in their private offices. Since nine out of ten couldn't pay, they were willing that public funds should pay them. They knew that somebody—aside from officials of the County Medical Society—must be responsible for and direct their death fight. The doctors asked to be made responsible to the city and county health officers. They faced the grim fact that—as in many another sickness—this dangerous disease often does not get to the doctor at all. More than half of the early—and most dangerous—syphilis never reached them!

"Damn it, there's all kinds of syphilis running round here *we* can't reach," said one family physician. "But we're going to find it and clean it out of the county." And they began the organization of a city venereal clinic.

V

When county medical societies—the nation over—become fired with the spirit of New York's and Michigan's doctors against pneumonia, and that of the Ingham County, Michigan, self-accusers against syphilis, the cancer death rate will not remain the national scandal it is today. Here again is material for medical self-accusation. Says a famous cancer specialist—

"The fate of the cancer patient is in the hands of the first physician that sees that patient."

So far as life or death goes, this is somewhat of an exaggeration, because some come with cancers impossible to get at, and incurable (even though still early) by the greatest of the world's cancer specialists. Of course it is to the family doctors that the majority of threatened people go. They are told to by growingly powerful publicity campaigns—urging them to see their doctors at first sign of chronic bleeding, or discharge from their bodies, of inside or outside sores that will not heal, of growing lumps, or moles that change color and begin to grow. Yet America's most distinguished cancer pathologist has said that the doctor—so slow to suspect cancer—is the greatest obstacle in driving down the cancer death rate.

Is this entirely the fault of the family doctor? He is untrained in cancer science. He feels he plays no effective part in the fight against this terror that kills eighty per cent of all its victims within four years after it is detected. And if tomorrow all doctors would suddenly become on the alert, instantly to suspect cancer, what would be the good of it . . . in wide areas of this country?

Over vast stretches, well-equipped and expertly staffed tumor clinics do not exist.

The New York State Health Department has surveyed the scandalous lack of weapons, of fighters to use them against this second most formidable of the killers of its people. The healthmen are now joining hands with the State Medical Society to try to stimulate physicians to organize tumor clinics in every general hospital worth the name. Here there must be modern x-ray apparatus, adequate radium, and an expert to use these more or less powerful but dangerous weapons safely. Such clinics must be staffed by doctors and pathologists skilled in diagnosis, by surgeons capable of the drastic operations that so often can save cancer sufferers' lives. These death-fighting teams must be directed by a new type of specialist—the cancer consultant.

But for most of upstate New York this project is a lovely dream, so far, because there is no money. Where tumor clinics are in operation—as in Dutchess County—the physicians are enthusiastic. Now they've somewhere to send their patients bombarded with propaganda "to see your doctor early." Here the practicing physicians are becoming cancer scouts for the specialists. At the new clinics the family doctors can follow the fascinating science of cancer diagnosis, the engineering of its modern treatment. And they give medical care to those patients who—alas—must suffer pain and discomfort from the heroic treatment that has a chance to save their lives. Becoming part of a cancer-fighting team, the doctor will see to it that his patients stick through their ordeal; he'll follow such patients, for years, to keep the records so necessary to prove whether or not they have maintained their cure.

After all, the most skilled surgery, the most powerful and expertly handled x-ray and radium treatment are at best only makeshift weapons against this great killer. If they were used with ideal skill on patients seen early enough, cancer fighters at New York's Memorial Hospital say one-third of cancer's victims could be saved. Can any community, with the wide lack of hospitals, laboratories, skilled medical care, hope to stem the steadily rising cancer death rate? Massachusetts has begun to do it. In this state quick diagnosis is in reach of all the state's doctors. There are two excellent hospitals for cancer treatment. The state's doctors teach the members of all kinds of civic groups, clubs, lodges, to see physicians early and they're actually cutting down—by months —the time from the ill's beginning to the first visit to the expert.

For the first time in any state's history, during the past two years the Massachusetts cancer death rate has not risen, but leveled off. The cancer death of women seems to begin to start downward. . . .

But everywhere the means to fight this curse are lacking. With moderate federal aid, doctors, officials of general hospitals, would leap into a public health fight against it. It is a murderous scandal that, today, there are general hospitals that discourage the installing of these tumor clinics. For cancer bears heavily upon the poor—and tumor clinics would attract poor people to the hospitals, which then would have to pay for the care of the chronic sufferers on their way to dying. This is the human condition of cancer victims in our rich America: that thousands of them must be turned away from hospitals, to be gnawed with their terminal pain, at home, and without nursing care. If general hospitals received aid in the housing of these far-gone wretches, they would welcome the organization of tumor clinics by their doctors— with the result that they'd have to house far fewer victims for whom all hope is gone.

The country's doctors are ready for this public health battle against cancer. They would join this battle, if only there were a modest amount of money to train cancer consultants, to pay physicians, alert to learn the rudiments of cancer science, for the time they take off from their practices to gain this life-saving knowledge. And they certainly deserve pay for the care of their cancer patients, and for the absolutely vital public health scouting out of early cancers, and for following the fate of those whose cure has been attempted.

For if the doctor is not worth his hire, then it is

folly to ask him to join the proposed national health army.

Till our federal government aids the states and communities in financing this hopeful death-fight, the present ballyhoo about cancer is only exquisite cruelty for those whose hopes are raised in vain—

For this is the infamy that mocks much of the see-your-doctor-early propaganda—

More than half of cancer's victims must go on being left to slow, horrible death *if paying for this fight for life is not made a public matter.*

VI

Since they took over this sacred duty from old wives and neighbor women, the most private, most personal toil of the family doctors was that of bringing new life into the world. This—till very recently —was only the mother's, the doctor's, and the baby's business. This was peculiarly sacred territory where public health did not enter. This, let's face it, was dark and bloody ground. Our healthmen, bookkeepers of life and death, could only record this grim fact: that, contrary to many descending death curves, the curve of dying of mothers and their new-born babies, held steady. Yet there existed known science to save mothers, and at last this good news got round to the people. Now, in the past few years it has become the people's demand that their physicians allow the healthmen onto this secret ground. Here and there—soon it will become nationwide—doctors are becoming their own maternal public healthmen.

In St. Lawrence County, New York—this is a vast rural region where child-bearing mothers could not be properly attended at home—the maternal and new-born infant death rates were scandalously high. 1933, Doctor Thomas Parran—then New York State Health Commissioner—stirred the St. Lawrence County Medical Society to study why so many of the county's new-born babies were dying. Out of this self-criticism came the doctors' demand that the country practitioners be aided by public health nurses —for bedside duty during childbirth. . . . So that somebody, skilled, would be on guard at all times during the mother's peril.

The nurses were supplied the doctors by the State Health Department. In 1936, the year before this simple aid of skilled vigilance was given the physicians, their shame was a maternal death rate of 8.4 per thousand live childbirths. 1937—that rate sank to 6.3. 1938—to 2.2, the lowest on record, far below the average maternal death rate for the nation. It shows brilliantly what modest measures—often—serve to dent the death rates, and what lives can be saved without in any way regimenting the doctors. All over New York state the county medical societies began to clean their own obstetric houses. The state's maternal death rate has gone down from 5.7 in 1936 to 3.5 per thousand live childbirths in 1938. Nationwide, maternal death is now down-trending, and this, again, is the cause of fanfare by the let-us-alone boys among the nation's physicians—

But for these let-us-alone complacent ones there is a hand-writing on the wall. For those medical politicos who view public accountability with alarm, this has been an argument, worked overtime: that rank-and-file physicians haven't the training, haven't got what it takes to bring death rates down to the ideal lows, called for by public health "fanatics." The medical politicos do not, of course, shout this from the housetops. They whisper it. This is the last stand of saboteurs of now possible life for the people. To this libel on the average doctor's ability the average doctor now arises to give the lie—

What your run-of-mine doctor can do to bring new life to mothers safely is now demonstrated at the Orange Memorial Hospital, at Orange, New Jersey. In this hospital, some eighty practicing physicians of the community deliver babies. To work here they must agree to one thing only: to submit themselves to supervision, at every childbirth if necessary, by skilled obstetricians. During something more than three years, they have delivered 3709 mothers—

Without a single obstetric maternal death! Compare this to the national rate of one out of two hundred!

Of course, despite everything that science can do, this wonderful record of safe childbirth will be marred finally. Physicians are—human. But these Orange, New Jersey, doctors have smashed the old alibi that in the matter of a mother's life you have to be—*too* human. Just like the Ingham County, Michigan, doctors in their fight against syphilis, these Orange birth-helpers are making medical history. Here is a spirit new in medical practice—expressed by the hospital's director, F. Stanley Howe—

"Our staff has gotten keyed up to such a point that it will go hard with the first doctor who loses a mother in our hospital."

But the hopeful angle of this spirit is that it is contagious, that it spreads to all those eighty doctors. Now when it "goes hard" it goes hard with the doctor's own estimate of himself if he loses a mother. "Teamwork and co-operation are important factors in our results," says F. Stanley Howe, "and our men spare no pains in giving a hand where one man has a difficult case, and you may believe me, we have had some pretty bad ones."

The example of this new spirit of the New York, Michigan, and New Jersey doctors is recommended for pondering by crackpots—and especially those in our federal government—who believe the way to raise the nation's health is by first of all antagonizing the doctors.

VII

Now the groundwork for a practical health program has been laid. It is now possible—nationwide —to clear up the misunderstanding between public healthmen and the doctors. The physicians ask only this assurance: that public healthmen—provided the doctors clean their own house—do not propose to steal their practices by unnecessary public clinics. It is the doctor who must treat the sick.

But in a really powerful national health program, the rank-and-file physicians cannot stop here. They can meet the public healthmen more than halfway. They can take far more advantage than they now do of this aid offered to them by healthmen—

The healthman's principal job is to see to it that physicians get into every home, not only to treat the sick, but to practice the new applied science of preventive medicine. Last Summer there was an infantile paralysis epidemic in Michigan. It was the public health authority—state and city—that broadcast by radio, newspapers, pamphlets that, in this epidemic season, every case of a child's feverish ailment—no matter how trivial—should immediately come under care of the family's doctor. This service by public healthmen vastly increased house calls by Michigan's doctors that 1939 Summer. Undoubtedly the doctors did prevent a great deal of serious crippling by spotting early cases of infantile paralysis and seeing to it that these children got the proper early treatment.

But how many of Michigan's doctors did what they could have done, in addition, when parents at the prodding of healthmen called the physicians into their homes?

In every one of these homes the doctor could be a public health detective. He could find out whether the children have received diphtheria and smallpox preventives. He could find out whether all the family have been tested for tuberculosis. . . . (Now he can advise periodic chest examinations for all the family by the new, highly accurate, ten cent x-ray micro-film that spots consumption in its first beginning.) . . . He can observe the state of nourishment of the children, and see if they are getting the proper life-giving vitamins and sunshine. In every family the doctor could be a nutrition expert—helping to prevent forms of heart disease, rheumatism, and, yes, insanity for which improper diet may, who knows, be in part to blame. For it begins to become clear that maximum nutrition will be the most powerful of all the life-guarding weapons of public health.

—It is here acknowledged that the physician, discovering families deteriorated, sick with this hidden hunger for vitamins, cannot be asked to buy them for the millions who themselves have not the wherewithal to feed strong life into their bodies. No, but the physician can become the chief social accuser of our political and financial leaders so murderously impotent to help the nation share its plenty—

Getting into these homes on his infantile paralysis mission, the practicing doctor's experienced eye can pick up clues of the beginning of wasting sicknesses. He can spot diabetes, thyroid trouble, cancer, heart disease—in fathers and mothers whom he's known in prime of health. Old fogeys may be horror-struck, saying this would be unethical, protesting that this would be drumming up business. But the people do not care a tinker's damn about medical ethics. They are no longer satisfied simply not to die, they do not propose to remain content with their doctor keeping them half alive. The people begin to grope for the strength, the defiance of the hard knocks of fate that can be brought by a full sap of life in their bodies. It is the family doctor who can begin to work for this new level of life, by carrying the still embryo science of it into every American home. This is the new responsibility of our physicians who are more and more brought into homes by our public healthmen. This is the now possible new opportunity, power, and glory that awaits the doctors.

VII. The People Demand Public Health *

THE PEOPLE of the United States intend to make their health a major concern of their government. This cannot be done unless the doctors are behind it. Today our physicians, as nationally organized, are still at outs with the federal government. No health program can get going till the government and the doctors stop squabbling and pull together.

These differences can be reconciled. Many physicians believe the federal government means to regiment them, to destroy their traditional private relation with their patients. It is true that an element among government planners has favored a health system that might endanger the independence of the doctors. Also, the Department of Justice has indicted officials of the American Medical Association.

The country's doctors feel themselves indicted, as a profession.

* Substantially as printed in *Country Gentleman*, January 1940.

Meanwhile, millions of our people go on need-lessly suffering. Hundreds of thousands needlessly die. The American people are the innocent bystand-ers. They are the victims of this childish doctor-government shindy. They will remain so till men of goodwill—from the science of medicine on the one hand and the federal government on the other—put an end to this frivolity of fighting over the bodies of the needlessly sick and dying people of our coun-try.

This is the gravest danger: unless the quarrel is soon settled, the people may cause enactment of health laws that will be wasteful, unworkable, and actually dangerous to the public health.

The American Medical Association has declared itself as opposed to the Wagner health bill, intro-duced in the Senate in 1939. But this does not mean that, as a profession, the doctors are opposed to all national health legislation, or that they consider a national health program impractical. In 1939, the House of Delegates of the American Medical Asso-ciation—the doctors' representative governing body —declared itself in favor of definite and decisive ac-tion on a national health law. Not sometime in the vague future. But *now*. In 1938 and 1939 Miss Roche's Interdepartmental Committee of health planners twice called a committee of seven physicians —appointed by the American Medical Association— into conference. These doctors state they were given no voice in the framing of the proposed health law. Their recommendations in no way influenced the framing of the Wagner health bill.

This has not been denied by any member of Miss Roche's Interdepartmental Committee.

Yet here is the hope for tomorrow's needlessly suffering and dying, here is the glory of our democracy: that no dictatorial government attempt has been made to ram health law down the throats of our physicians—who alone can make any health program effective. At public hearings, in Senate sub-committee on the Wagner health bill, the doctors had full fair chance to kick the daylights out of it. They did.

The question now arises: Can a sufficiently powerful element be found among our doctors—as nationally organized—to make practical, specific proposals of their own? And can government authority—other than the anti-doctor Roche Committee—be found to meet these physicians on common ground?

When you dig without prejudice through the 956 pages of the largely town-meeting talk of those Wagner health bill hearings, you find the American Medical Association physicians—though critical—

agree that the objects of the proposed law are not debatable. They also admit that a national health law could be made workable. You find the Senators conducting these hearings anxious to have the advice of the doctors. Many citizens have been misled by claims that opposition to the Wagner health bill is confined to a small clique of medical die-hards. "The enemies of this bill consist of a handful of reactionaries," said Mr. Lee Pressman, lawyer for the C.I.O. This was far from the case.

The Wagner health bill was criticized not only by officials of the American Medical Association, but by many progressive and distinguished physicians, by state health officers, and by no less than Thomas Parran, Surgeon General of the United States Public Health Service.

The President had asked his Interdepartmental Committee of health planners to co-ordinate the national activities in the fight for our health and lives. But all doctors and healthmen, testifying, agreed that the co-ordinators had failed to co-ordinate. Doctor Parran pointed out that the Wagner health bill lacked a unified plan. In fact, the bill further dispersed responsibility by setting up a new medical agency in social security. Under the proposed Wagner law, the fight for life would be scattered and overlapped among a lot of government bureaus, in the Public Health Service, the Department of Labor, the Social Security Board.

Our physicians and healthmen would, by this law, be forced to muddle about in a truly Russian tangle of red tape. The Department of Labor would help each state fight death of mothers and babies. The Public Health Service would help states down death rates from syphilis, cancer, tuberculosis, pneumonia, malaria, and preventable disease of people other than mothers and children. The Social Security Board—without medical personnel or experience—would try to take medical care of those Americans who are not mothers and babies, and who suffer from ills other than syphilis, tuberculosis, pneumonia, et cetera. Then still another bureau would be set up—to take special care of these various ills—of workingmen!

The entire bill, said Doctor Parran, was dominated by the special interests of labor and social insurance groups. Commenting on its chaotic proposals, Doctor Parran told the Senators: "We can never attain national health and fitness by making money grants to states out of several federal pockets."

Kentucky's famed health commissioner, Doctor Arthur T. McCormack, pictures the confusion into which the Wagner health bill, if enacted, might confound him—

"Think of Bill Jones on the creek having syphilis and his wife being pregnant, one of his children sick with an acute disease and another a crippled child, his grandfather paralyzed and his mother insane . . ."

While the dazed Health Commissioner McCormack himself cooled his heels in different government bureaus in Washington, begging for medical aid for the assorted unfortunates of the Jones family. While the Kentucky State Health Department had to send different doctors down the creek for each different disease and victim. While the people themselves suffered, while auditors and self-important government functionaries argued about who had authority over what, and where. It sounded highly soviet.

American Medical Association officials pointed out that the Wagner health bill did not safeguard the existence of the private practitioner. The Committee of Physicians, Inc.—rebels against the conservatism of the American Medical Association—agreed with Association officers that the proposed law would possibly increase the quantity of the medical care the American people were getting—but might actually damage its present quality. Hospital experts protested the vast sums proposed for building government hospitals without specific provision for aid of the excellent private but non-profit hospitals—financially distressed—now to be found all over the country. Doctor Parran made a final grave objection: the bill proposed appropriation of far too much money for the trained medical and public health men, now available to carry out the law's provisions.

In short, the Wagner health bill was the sort of abortion you'd expect from its framers who were essentially non-medical, not public healthmen—who had looked down their noses at medical and public health advice. It was plain that the Wagner health bill was not the answer to the people's demand for life and health.

I I

Yet from the Wagner bill hearings it was plain that our physicians and government healthmen—if they could only get together with all cards face up on the table—could now devise a sound, workable health law. What would be its basic principles?

The law must state its explicit intent that the federal government's part in a national health program is only that of giving money and technical aid—

where needed—to the states in their development of their own health programs, through sound scientific procedures.

The law must state that no plan approved under it shall provide for the regimentation, federalization of the practice of medicine. It must express its intent to provide in every possible way for the guarding of the present relation of doctors with their patients.

—Do health planners protest that this is succumbing to "organized medicine"? But who is competent to make us a healthy people? Our doctors or do-gooding crackpots?—

The national health law must be administered by one federal agency. This is already in existence. It is the U. S. Public Health Service—a highly competent, non-political force of physicians, trained in public health. This Service has a time-tried relationship with the health departments of all states. It has experience with programs of medical care. It bases its work and decisions on sound medical science, rather than upon political expediency. The Public Health Service does not dictate to state health services, and does not attempt to do so to doctors. It assists health agencies that can show need, and are competent according to scientific standards.

It is under this already existing force of physicians and healthmen that a national health program can be unified. There would have to be no setting up of a diversity of new government bureaus—for job-holding in these the Wagner health bill had proposed appropriation of over six million dollars, yearly!

To guard the needs and rights of every far-flung region in the country, and of the various basic medical disciplines, the Surgeon General—head of the national health program—should be supported by a council—or commission or committee or call it what you will—of distinguished physicians, scientists, and healthmen. These should have broad powers—more than advisory.

There should be a unified health authority in each state, guided again by a single council of physicians and healthmen. It is a disturbing fact that health commissionerships of the great majority of our states are political offices. They are not filled by scientific men appointed for competence only.

The new national health law must remedy this scandal. The federal government could limit its aid to those states with health commissioners appointed by a non-partisan health board of physicians and distinguished laymen. This board to be appointed by the governor, without regard to political party, and to serve overlapping terms. So the state health commissioner's job would no longer be a political football.

With these democratic and scientific controls, a health program could be written into law. A start could be made with what we've got right now. As Doctor Parran urges, the first steps should be taken in regard to those matters which are not controversial, and in regard to which there is great and obvious need.

Trusting the competence, sincerity, and goodwill toward the medical profession of Doctor Parran—and who rises to doubt these, who goes on record in public against them?—a committee of physicians can now join Doctor Parran in writing a practical health law. Its basic purpose would be not to take care of a sick America but to bring about a healthy America. It would immediately begin to expand the power of science against the killing and disabling diseases that can now be prevented. It would begin the establishment of ways and means to give medical care to every sick and suffering man, woman, and child in our nation who needs that care and does not now get it.

III

What would be the essentials of the titles of such a national health law if a national administration could ever be made to see the sense of sponsoring it, so that the Congress could be asked to pass upon it?

First and foremost, would be a title authorizing the public health agencies and the physicians of the United States to expand their already existing fight to control and wipe out the ills and deaths now preventable by known medical science. As it is now, this fight should be financed by state and local governments in so far as they can. It should be administered by them as it now is. But the fight would gain real power by technical and financial aid contributed by the federal government—acting through its health authority, the U. S. Public Health Service. The quicker these now controllable diseases and deaths are cut down, the less will be the present tremendous drain on the nation's pocketbook for mere medical care. The federal aid to the states should be experimental and flexible, with no long range vast spending plans as advocated in the Wagner health bill. At the present time the long or costly or only partly effective fights against pneumonia, syphilis,

gonorrhea, tuberculosis, malaria, pellagra, are becoming—thanks to new and rapidly evolving discoveries—not only immensely more powerful, but vastly
cheaper.

IV

But a national health program cannot stop with
prevention. The second title of such a law should certainly deal with ways and means to help our physicians care for the immense amount of sickness in our
nation that is inadequately treated or not treated at
all. This is also economic. Well-trained doctors and
nurses can do something to shorten disability from
rheumatic and nervous ailments. They can possibly
lengthen the lives of victims of heart and blood ves-
sel disease. They already do this for the lucky few
who can pay for truly adequate medical care. They
could do it for all Americans—

With a health law that would justly spread the
terrible individual burden of medical care, a law that
would see to it that our doctors could give this care
without being turned into government jobholders
and robots. This must be done by the doctors themselves. Federal welfare agencies such as the Social
Security Board, and other welfare agencies, state

and local, have no medical knowledge, less medical judgment, and even less medical discrimination. When welfare organizations hire physicians to the poor, ninety-nine times out of a hundred they are poor physicians. It is the contention of our wisest medical leaders, and of Doctor Thomas Parran, that universal medical care can be organized by the private physicians themselves, in co-operation with public healthmen.

Any health law aiding the doctors of our localities and states to care for the indigent only, would but scratch the surface of today's medical neglect of millions of Americans. So costly are the weapons of today's powerful medical science—the doctor's bill is only a small part of these services—that a serious chronic illness in fairly well-off families of our middle income brackets makes these families *medically indigent*. Though they are well able to pay their own way in the matter of food, clothing, shelter, fuel—and transportation. There are millions of such families today trying to balance their marginal budgets by neglect of their health, in the words of Doctor Parran.

How can a national health law help our physicians to meet this vast, disseminated disaster? The doctors have been trying to cope with it by charity—which

Americans hate—estimated at a total of more than a million dollars' worth of free treatment, daily. But how can a national health law help the physicians to provide medical care for the vast American mass, not only the relief and works program people, but the millions in the low and middle income brackets?

How can this be done? Not by herding millions of sick folks—under a system of compulsory insurance —into clinics where they get so-so care from an overworked salaried physician who must see about a hundred patients a day to earn his meager salary of around three thousand dollars a year!

This can be done by letting all citizens walk with shoulders straight into the office of a doctor or group of doctors they can choose themselves—to get adequate medical care, as good care as the next man, the care that's the fifth human right, as much of a right as the right to food, shelter, clothing, and fuel.

Many independent groups of doctors are organizing, with groups of citizens, to spread the burden of medical and hospital care. In California, in New Jersey, the state organizations of physicians are experimenting. The doctors of the Michigan State Medical Society believe they have found the answer. Medical service plans, such as theirs already in action, could under the new health law be aided by the federal health authority.

For nine years this progressive and public-spirited organization of Michigan's physicians has become more and more disgusted with the infamy of Michigan's millions, sick without money to buy decent medical and hospital care. These physicians did not pose as altruists. They were impatient, too, at doing a good one-third of their work with no pay for it. Headed by Detroit's Doctor Henry A. Luce, for nine years the Michigan State Medical Society has had its experts studying every known plan for health insurance, compulsory as well as voluntary.

Now they have taken action. For adequate medical care of all Michigan's people in middle and low income brackets—the people want that care or can be taught to want it—Michigan's doctors have organized a voluntary, non-profit corporation. This is the Michigan Medical Service. Every licensed physician in the state can belong to it. State law has been passed, enabling it. A board of directors, composed of physicians and laymen, administers it. The State Insurance Department supervises it. What will it do for Michigan's sick people?

Families with incomes of $2500 and under, or individuals with maximum income of $2000, organizing themselves into groups of not less than 25, can obtain medical care from doctors of their own choice. Employers can contribute part of the cost to help employees obtain the benefits of this plan. The Ford Motor Company has already joined it—on behalf of its more than eighty thousand employees. As this is written, though the plan has only been in operation for a few months, over 150,000 Michigan people are clamoring to get in under Michigan Medical Service.

The maximum yearly payment, for a family, for this service, is $54. This entitles the family to home and office medical care and to hospital visits by their doctors—to an extent of $875. In parallel the hospitals of the state have organized a group hospital service, for care at a yearly cost of $24 per family.

But what of the masses of Michigan's people without the necessary $78 per family for medical and hospital care? Michigan Medical Service has organized a medical relief division. For those indigent or in low income groups, arrangement may be made with local, state, or governmental agencies for them to pay part or all of the subscription cost. The poor family can receive unlimited medical care, every service the doctor of medicine can render in home, office, or hospital. For the care of these people the Michigan doctor will receive approximately half of his usual fee. The welfare agencies will pay the doctors for this service at the modest cost of forty cents per month per capita of the low income and relief population.

The physicians of Ingham County, Michigan— you recall their public-spirited fight against syphilis? —have already put this plan into action for all the indigent of that county. They have, in short, as a county-wide organization of physicians, taken action in the matter of the fifth human right. Again, as in their self-criticism on their failure to act as public healthmen against syphilis, they are making medical history.

What then would be the federal government's part in aiding doctors of states organizing medical group service for all citizens who cannot pay for adequate medical service individually? Under a national health law, the federal health authority would make grants to such states as cannot by themselves bear the total cost of their statewide medical care of their people in those income brackets where any serious or chronic sickness means financial disaster.

This is a big country and every state's resources, and its medical needs, are different. But Michigan's medical care plan can be made flexible enough to meet the needs of all American localities. Every state will have to cut and try, in the matter of what income brackets should be included in its group medical service plan, what subscription rates can be borne by its people, what part will have to be paid by public agencies, what fees are fair to its doctors. A national health law that encouraged compulsory health insurance in any state would be sure to antagonize the doctors. It would be sabotaged by them. On the other hand, if a national health law explicitly encouraged every state's doctors to work out their own voluntary group medical service system, the doctors will go on giving medical care while the bookkeeping details of the voluntary group insurance system are being worked out.

Michigan's doctors have been in the dog-house with high medico-politicians for their pioneering effort in spreading the burden of medical care. But medical moss-backism cannot stop these progressive physicians in their fight to lead the people toward this fifth human right.

V

In addition to aiding the doctors and healthmen of the states to prevent disease and give medical care to all the people, the national health law will have to make provision for aid to hospitals, wherever state or local finances cannot meet the needs. More and more, as medical science triumphs over disease and death, our hospitals, with their technical equipment for diagnosis and cure, are becoming the heart of the fight for life. First of all, the national health law should provide for aid to states in assisting in maintaining and properly equipping those voluntary, non-profit, charitable and religious hospitals that already exist. It is a tragic fact that today hundreds of thousands of hospital beds are empty. Not because there are no sick to fill them. Not because hospital authorities are stony-hearted. But because our hospitals cannot afford to take care of more sick people free of charge. And many existing hospitals are miserably equipped and staffed for today's fights against cancer, syphilis, rheumatism, mental illness and other diseases. A national health law should bring these strong points against death to top death-fighting power. It should see to it that present hospital beds are available to the people, according to the needs of the various states and localities. The same holds true for all public hospitals—particularly those for the treatment of tuberculosis and mental diseases.

But even after this has been accomplished there are regions, especially rural, where there is a murderous deficit of modern hospitals, where there are no hospitals or laboratory-health centers at all. It is up to the citizens of these regions—through their physicians and healthmen—to make these needs known to the federal health authority that will be charged with aiding the states under a national health law. And while the rural need for hospitals is outstanding, many large cities suffer actual shortage of hospital beds. This is scandalously true today of Baltimore —one of the greatest medical centers in the country.

There are preventable deaths—notably tuberculosis—which many states cannot even begin to fight effectively till the present lack of TB sanatoria is remedied. This can only be done on a nationwide basis by federal aid.

V I

Even with amply available hospital beds, with the latest gadgets against death, with the most elaborate laboratories—our physicians and healthmen could not even then turn on the real power of today's science. Until they have the opportunity to keep abreast of its constant development, keep up to the minute on how to use its mighty, expanding arsenal of weapons against death. Our physicians make about

$3000 a year, on the average. It is absolutely out of the question to ask them to take time off from their practices, and to spend the money to go back, each year or every two years, to some medical school for the needed postgraduate training.

Yet their knowledge becomes obsolete much faster than do automobiles. Even young doctors, not more than five years out of medical school, blunder dangerously with the powerful new life-saving chemicals sulfanilamide and sulfapyridine, and with the new super-charged hormones. The Committee of Physicians, Inc.—revolting against medical moss-backism—points out that medical education is far more expensive and time-consuming than any other form of learning. The medical schools and other medical teaching institutions today can't even meet their proper obligations to the students studying for their M.D.'s—let alone take on the burden of the desperately necessary postgraduate teaching of doctors. In the new health army to be organized under a national health law, high standards of competence will be demanded of the fighters. But what's the use of setting up such standards, when there's no way for doctors to meet those standards?

So the new national health law must make explicit provision to aid the states in giving all their doctors, public healthmen, laboratorians, nurses, periodic study courses to keep them posted, to enable them to use new death-fighting weapons. It must aid the scientists now baffled in their researches for lack of death-fighting money. Particularly, federal aid is necessary for the medical schools. For the burden of sickness and death will never be lifted from the American people's shoulders until the medical schools are open to the highest type of aspiring young men and women, no matter whether they are well-off or poor—

In contrast to the present method of recruiting raw material for doctors, on the principle that the aspirant for an M.D. must have a well-heeled father. Government dollars spent for fellowships to pick out the very highest type of young Americans—as we do for the Army and Navy at West Point and Annapolis— would be repaid many times over. If we can pay for the education of our best youth to kill humanity, we can afford to train the best to save human life.

VII

The fundamental principle of the new national health program is expressed in three one-syllable words: Health is wealth. But this must be proved in dollars and cents. That means the new national health law must make provision for an absolutely new kind of men against death. These are public health accountants. These experts will set up a new kind of national bookkeeping. Their investigations will establish the costs of disease and death to the nation—of every kind of ill and death. It will keep tab on how federal and state moneys are being spent to fight all disease and death. It will demonstrate wasteful expenditures to the taxpayers. It will set up a new giant balance sheet. This will account for the nation's sickness and death in red ink; and for the savings—now possible by human conservation—in black. It will be a cost-accounting of life and death in terms of dollars. It will prove that funds properly spent for medical care and disease prevention are sound money investments for the nation. It has been claimed that the vast sums now spent for work relief, for conservation of soil and forests, even for defense will ultimately pay themselves off as investments for more wealthy future America. But our new public health accountants could prove the financial soundness of money spent for human conservation—with far greater accuracy. If only the health program under the new health law is financed as a long-range, self-liquidating project.

VIII

These are the essentials of a workable health law, not revolutionary, but beginning with the medical, public health, scientific, and banking men and institutions that exist right now.

The people—when it's put to a vote—want this fight for their lives. Even when it means a temporary drain on their pocketbooks—never heavy compared to other taxes—they demand it. In Michigan this was demonstrated by a poll recently taken by the W. K. Kellogg Foundation. For some time this Foundation has maintained full time health units in seven Michigan counties. For some nine years, now, these units have been in operation—working closely with the physicians and the public. Last year the Foundation asked the tax-paying citizens, in a straw ballot, whether they would now help maintain this health service, to the extent of an annual twenty-five cents *per capita* of the people?

The number who voted, who returned the ballots mailed to them, is the highest ever heard of in any poll taken in our country. Their answer was unmistakable—

65,338 in these seven Michigan counties voted

"Yes." Only 863 voted against the proposed assessment to help maintain their county health units.

And, nationwide, wherever such full time health units have helped physicians in their fight for the lives of the people, the citizens never fail to retain them—even when county finances are made low as they have been in our economic tailspin.

Now the fight for life can extend from counties to the nation—if the now possible practical health law is enacted. Those who will administer its above outlined five titles are ready to do so. The United States Public Health Service and the State Health Departments are ready to expand the fight against preventable disease and death. The doctors, as organized in counties and states, are ready to direct the spreading of the burden of the medical care of the people. Federal works agencies and private building industry are all set to build the hospitals, health centers, and laboratories needed—if the federal government will aid them. Authorities who run existing voluntary and public hospitals know exactly what they need to maintain and expand the death-fighting power of their institutions—if government and state aid becomes available. The faculties of medical schools and public health agencies can rapidly organize the postgraduate teaching of the nation's physicians and public healthmen, laboratorians, and nurses. They could quickly design, too, a system of fellowships for poor but able young men and women who should have the opportunity to join the new health army. The financial leaders of the country could show our political leaders how the new public health-accounting division of the federal health authority could be set up, and could demonstrate where the nation could get the money to finance its program of human conservation.

What then delays us?

VIII. Death Does Not Wait

NOW AGAIN it was autumn at Wake Robin, but there was not the hopelessness about getting action for human conservation, there was not now the despair that had made the 1938 Autumn so gloomy. Cy Young was right. The stories telling how public health was good for doctors, how public health needed them, both struck fire, and while they were still in manuscript, before publication.

Doctor L. G. Christian, of Lansing, Michigan, read them, and proceeded to set wheels in motion. Greg Christian was one of those physicians with an ear tuned to the growing muttering of the demand of the people for health, for life. He saw the writing on the wall warning the nation's doctors against medical moss-backs whose answer to this popular demand was only a petulant "let us alone."

Christian trusted the competence of Doctor Thomas Parran as a public health leader. He believed in Parran's good will toward the doctors of the nation. He agreed with Parran—that the American public is not the doctor's oyster, that the doctors are servants of the American people, and that the people have as good a right to state the terms under which they wish to have medical care, as the doctors have a right to blueprint the conditions under which they will give it.

Mind you, Greg Christian was no medical rebel, was what is called "regular." He was convinced that the physicians, through their organizations, could spread the fifth human right to the people. But he knew they'd get nowhere without the public health-men, and that they needed state and federal governmental aid. In short, Christian was realistic. He was sacrificing his practice, fighting for this fifth human right as one of the five members of the Michigan State Social Welfare Commission. Among the doctors he was one of the boys, but if the doctors refused to join in fights to cut down the death rates, let's say, of cancer, then Christian admitted cancer would have to be fought in public clinics. . . .

Though often roughly outspoken and certainly no Henry Clay type of compromiser, yet Christian believed the government and the doctors could be got together. Christian offered to demonstrate the good will of doctors by arranging a little conference for me with three of Michigan's medical leaders. This was an illuminating experience. This meeting was dominated by kindly and distinguished Doctor Henry A. Luce, Past-President of the Michigan State Medical Society, and a veteran member of the House of Delegates of the American Medical Association. Luce picked his words, in a precise way of talking, giving news of the sentiment among a large section of those high in national medical councils. It was heartening. It was surprising in view of the widely broadcast anti-governmental medical defiance.

Luce explained what the public didn't know, what Doctor Parran himself didn't realize—that when the doctors' House of Delegates had held their famous special session at Chicago in September, 1938, and had gone on record as favoring action, *now*, on a health program, they hadn't meant maybe. This had been a truly democratic meeting. The delegates led the meeting. They voted down an attempt to limit their debates. "Never before in the history of the House did the delegates assume such leadership," says Doctor T. K. Gruber, who as a delegate was there, and should know. The official declarations of that session were no rubber-stamping of a handout gotten up beforehand by what is damned as "the medical hierarchy." Committees of public-spirited doctors had worked, day and night, batting out those momentous resolutions that held out the olive branch to the government. They refused to be stooges for a coterie of big boys who might try to run the shebang from a "little smoke-filled room."

But here, explained Luce, was the rub: the committee of seven physicians, appointed by this House of Delegates meeting to co-operate with the government, when they got to Washington, got what was in effect the bum's rush from Josephine Roche's health-planning brain-trusters. Luce had been one of these seven doctors, and he knew. The doctors were treated politely—but they were shown that this was merely a "hearing," not a conference with them treated as equals. Then on top of this snub had come the government indictment of the five officials of the American Medical Association. Now these officials, said Luce, had only been interpreting the actions of the House of Delegates, the A.M.A.'s governing body. "I, for one, feel that as a physician, personally, I have been indicted by the U. S. government. . . . The . . . reflection upon the integrity of the American Medical Association is considered by me as a reflection upon myself," said Luce.

In short, he felt the smear had been put on the

doctors in America. And did the people believe for one minute that 113,000 docs were—criminals?

Now Luce came down to brass tacks. Maybe the defiant element of the American Medical Association were right about believing they'd lick the government in this lawsuit, hands down. But what about the people who were sick, who were dying? They were caught in the middle. It was, said Luce, to the nation's interest that neither side win this silly lawsuit!

This was thrilling. It would be an eye-opener for would-be medical socializers who considered our physicians as nationally organized to be a camorra of rogues and tories. Henry Luce and his companions at this present little conference—Doctor Henry R. Carstens and Doctor A. S. Brunk—were no medical radicals. They were middle-of-the-roaders, medical liberals, in no sense pinkos. But the three of them were responsible men. Carstens was Chairman of the Council of the Michigan State Medical Society and Brunk was a council member. It was plain that the three of them were looking for a way to tell Uncle Sam that, if he wanted it, they could offer him the cordial co-operation of a majority of the nation's physicians. . . .

Luce explained to me that he was fed up with dirty grapevine medical insinuations—never openly made—that Surgeon General Thomas Parran was some sort of medical communist. "If I'd been in Parran's position in all this argument," said Luce, "there isn't a thing he has said or done that I would have said or done differently."

Could a meeting with Doctor Parran be arranged?

Would it do any good to tell Parran that there were men of good will in medicine who wanted that silly suit against the doctors to be settled? Would it interest Parran to know that the old olive-branch committee of seven physicians had never been dismissed? That it would really be willing to co-operate with the government toward a workable health program?

I said it was pretty certain that the meeting could be arranged. And it was held in Detroit, October 14, 1939. It was memorable, if you still had faith in our funny democracy, in the existence of plenty of American men of high competence and good will who were disgusted with the people's needless dying. That night all cards were face up on the table between Thomas Parran and the Michigan doctors. Parran was modest as always—"only a little man in Washington"—and said he was not to be considered as speaking for the government high command. On their part the Michigan physicians let

Parran feel they had faith in him as a government officer anxious to serve the country's people and doctors alike. And they wanted right now to lay a plan on the line—

Doctor Thomas K. Gruber—like Luce and Christian a member of the A.M.A.'s House of Delegates —was there this evening. Gruber is the kind of hombre no wise man gets gay with. He was outspoken against medical moss-backism and is known, in medico-political circles, as a hatchet man for progressive medicine. "I have this comment to make," said Gruber, "if the doctors and the public of this country don't look out, somebody is going to get burned. . . . This business of calling bad names and setting up destructive criticism gets everybody interested nowhere fast."

Greg Christian outlined to Doctor Parran Michigan's group medical care plan for its people in low income brackets and all those on welfare and work relief. He was proud it was now ready for action. With Henry Luce, Christian had been one of a group who'd worked for nine years to put this fifth human right over. What Michigan's doctors had now officially done, every state medical organization could do. . . . And, yes, would do, if only the government—

It was one of those human gatherings unforget-able because here you see six egos merging into com-mon understanding, into unanimity that leads to action.

Now Thomas Parran asked the Michigan doctors —Henry A. Luce, Thomas K. Gruber, L. G. Chris-tian, Henry R. Carstens, and A. S. Brunk—to draw up a memorandum. This to embody *their* ideas of a practical, workable national health law. Parran would then present this memorandum to his su-periors at Washington. If they were impressed with it, then maybe that committee of seven physicians, from the American Medical Association, would again be called to Washington. . . . Not this time to be given the high hat. . . . But as for those indict-ments, Parran was by no means sure that anything could be done about them or whether it was worth while to try to do anything about them.

It is to the credit of the group of Michigan physi-cians, that evening, that they did not make the settle-ment of this government lawsuit against the A.M.A. officials a condition for their co-operation on a memo-randum for a health law. It was enough, for them, that one government man, Parran—whom they trusted though he could make no promises at all—

had asked them to draw up constructive recommendations.

The Michigan doctors told Parran they'd get right to work on this job, and the meeting broke up very late that night in an atmosphere of comradeship, of determination, and hope.

Here, verbatim, is the memorandum, the result of the work in October and November, 1939, of Doctors Luce, Carstens, Brunk, Christian, and Gruber—unanimous.

II

Fundamental Principles of a Non-controversial National Health Program.

(1) The basic purposes of a national health law are: (a) federal aid to the states to expand activity against disease and death now wholly or in part controllable or preventable by now known and available medical science, and

(b) federal aid to the states in establishing sound ways and means to make available medical care to the medically indigent of the nation; medically indigent are those who are unable, in the place where they reside, through their own resources, to provide themselves and their dependents with proper medical, dental, nursing, hospital, pharmaceutical, and

therapeutic-appliance care without depriving them-selves or their dependents of necessary food, cloth-ing, and similar necessities of life, as determined by the local authorities dispensing relief for the medi-cally indigent. This establishes the fifth human right, the right of medical care, in addition to the rights to food, clothing, shelter, and fuel now recognized.

(2) The law must state that the federal govern-ment's part in a national health program is only that of giving money and technical aid—where needed and when requested—to the states in their develop-ment of their own health programs through sound and scientific procedures of their own choice. The duly constituted authority of the federal government shall set up minimum standards for these procedures.

(3) The health law must explicitly state that no plan approved under it shall provide for the regi-mentation or federalization of the practice of medi-cine. It must provide in every way for safeguarding the relationship of patient and doctor as now existing in private practice.

(4) The law must be administered by a unified federal agency. It is proposed that this agency be a U. S. Public Health department, which will unify all existing governmental medical and health activi-ties—excepting those of the Army and Navy—in one organization. This department to be organized along the lines of the U. S. Public Health Service, which has a time-tried relationship with the Health De-

partments of all states, which does not act upon political expediency, and which carries out sound health programs in conformity with the accepted principles of the science of medicine.

(5) The administration of the health program shall be locally determined by the various states in co-operation with the medical profession of the respective states.

(6) The federal health program should only provide facilities for those who render the service in order that the highest type of service be available to all. The federal health program should in no manner render the actual service as regards the care of the sick.

(7) The federal health program shall in no manner whatsoever provide for, make possible, or grant support to any compulsory type of health insurance or compulsory medical service insurance.

Paragraphs (1) to (7) inclusive, above, state the general principles of a health program. Below is stated the substance of possible titles of the bill which might be enacted into health law with a minimum of controversy.

(8) The first title of the national health law shall provide for financial and technical aid to the various states in their programs of preventive medicine, by the federal health authority—in those instances where the states can show need—according to a uniform and equitable national standard.

(9) *The second title of the national health law shall provide for federal financial aid to the various states—where need can be shown according to a uniform and equitable national standard—for the medical care of those who are medically indigent as defined in paragraph (1) (b), above. The programs for the medical care of the medically indigent shall be worked out, co-operatively, by the medical profession and the public of each state. Such programs shall not disturb the private physician-patient relationship. Such programs can best be based on the organization of pre-payment, non-profit group medical care plan to which federal funds may be allocated to supplement state and local funds—where need can be shown according to uniform and equitable national standards.*

(10) *The third title of the national health law shall provide for federal financial and technical aid in maintaining and supplying technical equipment to publicly owned hospitals and at the same time to those voluntary, non-profit, charitable, and religious hospitals and laboratories that already exist. It shall provide aid for the construction and aid in maintenance of hospitals and laboratories in regions—particularly rural ones—which lack such institutions. This construction and maintenance of new facilities to be federally aided only in those regions of states where the medical profession and hospital adminis-*

*trations and civic groups can show that already exist-
ing facilities are not being duplicated or replaced.*

(*11*) *The fourth title of the national health law
shall provide for federal aid to the states—where
need can be shown according to a uniform and equitable national standard—in keeping the physicians,
public healthmen, laboratorians, and nurses abreast
of our constantly developing medical science. It may
provide aid to accredited laboratories and medical institutions in the states—where need can be shown according to uniform and equitable national standards
—for research directed toward improving means of
treating and controlling diseases now in part controllable, and toward finding means for treatment
and control of diseases for which scientific means for
treatment and control do not now exist. It may provide, finally, for aid to accredited medical schools in
the states—where need can be shown according to
uniform and equitable national standards—in the
education of the highest type of young men and
women who aspire to the profession of medicine, regardless of economic status. Only by such improvement in medical education and research can a national health program insure improvement in quality
of preventive medical service and of medical care.*

(*12*) *The fifth title of the national health law
must make explicit provision for a new medical and
public health function: that of public health and
medical accounting. Such an actuarial function cannot*

223

only provide knowledge of the cost of disease to the nation, but it can keep constant tab on how federal and state moneys are being spent for the prevention of disease. It can demonstrate wasteful expenditures to the taxpayers. In the long view it can prove that the funds properly spent for the prevention of disease and for medical care are the soundest of all possible national investments. For it is axiomatic that it costs more to maintain disease in a nation than it costs to control it. The best assurance to taxpayers against money-waste in a health program is to set up such a program as a long-range, self-liquidating project.

III

To keep the promise made to Doctor Luce, a conference was now arranged and held with Attorney General Frank Murphy, on November 1, 1939. Mr. Murphy had not initiated, he explained to us, but had, rather, inherited the government lawsuit against the officials of the American Medical Association. He further explained that everybody and his brother from all over the country was constantly coming to him wanting Federal indictments dismissed, for more or less good reasons. He had been informed that, in spite of reverses, the government was sure to win the lawsuit ultimately. But then

Henry Luce—as always picking his words with precision—proved to the Attorney General that it was to the American people's interest that neither side triumph in this legal shindy. Murphy saw the point of it. He explained that in his opinion, the right of the people to medical care and to maximum health was not the fifth, but the first, of all human rights. And that if this doctor-medical quarrel could be viewed as a minor event in the major project of a great national program of human conservation, then something *might* be done about it—

Now such a momentous matter lay outside and above his own personal authority and powers. But he would be glad to urge action for nationwide human conservation to the President. . . .

After two years of frustration, was there now at last going to be a chance to paint the picture of the possibilities of a national health program to the President? Frank Murphy was a powerful friend at court. Now, too, Howard Hunter believed it inconceivable that the President would not be deeply interested in a practical non-controversial health program. Like Murphy he was a man to keep promises and with a record of action for the people's health.

So now from the White House came the call to me for this conference—for December 13, 1939. It is curious how a coming event—that you've been dreaming about and wangling for—when it looms as a reality, now worries and frightens you. It must be what challengers feel like when they know that, next week, they're going to have a crack at the heavy-weight championship. Now I never felt a doubt about the soundness of the plan for human conservation, the rightness of the thesis that health is wealth. It was not a matter of lack of personal confidence in it. I felt absolutely confident in taking it to the President because it was the product of the brains, the technical competence, the experience, the devotion of Henry Vaughan, Pat O'Brien, Bruce Douglas, Bill Scripps, Max Peet, Karl Meyer, Bill Lorenz, Doc O'Connor, Tom Parran, O. C. Wenger, Herman Bundesen, George Woods, Phil Rose, Dave Noyes, Henry Luce, Greg Christian, Henry Carstens, Andy Brunk, Tommy Gruber, and good old Cy Young—

This gang were one, back of you, and they couldn't be wrong. And yet there remained personal misgivings about power to present the desirability, the necessity of the health program—now that the great chance had come—to the one man who really could say yes or no.

Dave Noyes was now a tower of strength for me. That little bundle of public-relations sagacity, of energy, of complete lack of awe of overpowering personalities, now gave me heartening counsel. There was no use to go asking the President for half a loaf for public health, said Noyes, but there was only one thing to do: to go all out. You'd get nowhere piddling timidly around about it. The President must be made to see the situation was ripe for action, that he alone could underwrite this greatest of all public causes, about which there'd been too much delay and haggling, already. The public has been caught in too many places—as in Chicago, for example—between dirty local politics and a narrow guild spirit of mossback doctors. With the public-spirited physicians now ready to back a practical health program, the President, sponsoring a national health law, could expose and clean out these enemies of the people. . . .

Now Dave Noyes warmed up to his subject. Here was what to tell the man in the White House. In the past six years, Mr. President, you have dramatized the material misery of the lower economic levels. But the tragedy of a man out of a job—but who can still pound the pavements—is not to be compared with the tragedy of mass sickness and death, in the face of today's existing life-saving science. You, as a human being, Mr. President, are concerned for what posterity will think of you. Remember the rich men

—even the modern robber barons—who have bought themselves enduring respectability by their endowments of medical schools, hospitals, laboratories. . . . How much greater a monument is now ready to be built, if you'll lead the whole nation to concentrate its might, its tremendous resources on a program of human conservation. . . . The start should be modest, while the health army is trained and mobilized, but the start is everything, and only you can give us the green light. Look at Pasteur. His own actual life-saving was negligible. But the life-saving, accumulating for fifty years post-Pasteur and because of him, is the greatest of all steps forward in human history. Now the supercharging by a national human conservation program, of the fight for life of which our physicians and healthmen are capable and which the people demand—what other stroke of statesmanship could compare with it? You are dedicated, Mr. President, to the perpetuation of your humane policies, whether or no you remain at the national helm. Now consider a real program of human conservation. It is not controversial. It can and should be supra-political. Yet it is the most powerful of all political weapons. It should be made the cornerstone of all your plans for a happier America. In this war-mad world, the public health program can be made a rider to the issue of national defense—that being now an issue on which there is no serious disagreement. Who denies that the nation's health is the first line of defense? And you can guard your health program from being made a political football. Prominent men of the opposite persuasion in politics are vitally interested in human conservation. For them, on this issue, all political barriers will be down. They'd join a coalition for the lives of the people. Look at the way, Mr. President, that *Country Gentleman* has developed and stood back of this human conservation program. Yet this is certainly no pro-New Deal publication. But for this conservative mass circulation periodical there have been no politics on this issue. . . . You have been savagely criticized as the enemy of private enterprise. If you now take action for a healthy nation, you take action for an independent citizenry. As father of a program of human conservation you would lift the energy of America's people. And what is private enterprise but personal energy?

And, finally, in this land with new race hatred ominous, and menaced from abroad and at home by communazi threats to our democracy, common action for the public health would be the greatest of all—integrators. . . .

Such was the argument that came like a torrent out of fighting Dave Noyes. And would to God he had been instead of myself the man to be detailed to carry this story to the President. He should have been.

There is a peculiarity about conferring with the President—it is not the man but awe of the dignity of his office—there is this that makes it not exactly a man-to-man, a fifty-fifty conversation—

You go armed to tell him, but if he has his own ideas, he tells *you*. And you listen.

So, this 13th of December, 1939, Dave Noyes's argument did not get told. Or only fragments of it.

From this conference it was clear that the President was interested, yes, in the public health. But—and this is the most terrible little word in our language—but this was not the time to begin a large-scale health program. The President had his own plan for building hospital health centers in rural regions that needed them. But a general human conservation program for all the country? In view of the heavy demands now made on the nation's financial resources by the need for national defense?

For a health program, where would you get the money? So it was no use to present the memorandum on a non-controversial health law that I had brought hopefully to this conference in an inside coat pocket. . . .

IV

It was a personal failure, a defeat, that the picture of the power and the glory of human conservation could not be told by word of mouth, man-to-man, to the President. No alibi is here presented. There was an element of buck fever about it, yes. It was like a palooka prize-fighter getting flustered when the bell for the first round rings, and then for the rest of the fight forgetting the advice of his trainer. . . .

So that's that. So no nationwide program of human conservation will be launched in 1940. So it's best to remember Tom Parran, who is always talking about the long haul. So human conservation—which could be and should be the spearhead of human progress—is not for right now, maybe? Well, there is always the typewriter to go back to. This is a free country, with no Gestapo or Ogpu to take you for a ride for saying what you think, for writing what you know is true.

Yes, there was Wake Robin and the typewriter to go back to. After all, in our democracy it is the people who really are the President. In the long run the President is only the servant who must execute the people's will. There are years ahead. There will be other Presidents. There must come a President forced to take action, when at last the demand of the people for life becomes strong enough, and united.

Out of the frustrations of the past five years' battle for nationwide human conservation, there is a residue of hope, there is some good news to tell. The people can be truly told that the doctors of the country—as nationally organized—are now ready to take leadership in a national health program.

The three stories about the doctors' part in public health—published in expanded form in this present book as Chapters V, VI, and VII—were advertised to the nation's doctors, for free distribution by the *Country Gentleman,* early in 1940. The response of the physicians was generous and strong.

With the support of our best medical leaders, and with pressure upon our political leaders by a powerful "people's health lobby" which there is now hope of organizing, it is probable that within a few years the beginning of a national health program will be enabled by federal law. But national saving of money by saving lives is only the first phase of this program of human conservation. There are medical leaders who already see beyond this sordid reason for a national fight for life.

The people can take courage from the stir in the ranks of their physicians. They have gone on record as being ready to take their place as pioneers in a nationwide advance toward a higher level of life which the people are already demanding. This advance will not be dictated by spurious political promises, or by any well-intentioned but unreliable spirit of do-gooding. It will be guided by the power of medical science.

The country's doctors—as nationally organized—have thus placed themselves on record in one of their major criticisms of the Wagner health bill. In regard to this, the report of the reference committee of the House of Delegates of the American Medical Association, May, 1939, stated—

"The Wagner bill does not recognize the need for suitable food, sanitary housing, and the improvement of other environmental conditions necessary to the continuous prevention of disease and to health."

There you have the doctors themselves saying, about the myriads in our lower economic levels—

What's the use of our saving the lives of mothers in childbirth, what's the use of our bringing sound babies into the world, what's the good of our curing

233

the sick and suffering as we now can do, what's the good of our preventing disease—just to see the people kept half-alive, subsisting as millions of them now do, on food not fit for dogs to eat, in houses not fit for swine to inhabit.

This new spirit of the science of medicine is the best of news for the people. This is the science of medicine coming of age. The power of science now brings new life safely to American mothers living in the worst of slums. Just let all fathers and mothers realize this. Then the contrast of the beauty and power of that science on the one hand and the desolation of the slums on the other—will make those slums ridiculous to the people, will make them no longer tolerable.

So our men of medical science are ready to open up a new frontier in our nation. It is an internal frontier. It means the razing of our country and the building of our country over—which alone will allow the people to live at a level of health and vigor that our new medical science can give them.

Our doctors—alone competent to furnish the scientific basis for it—stand ready to help our engineers, industrialists, builders, and workers to draw up the blueprints for a new America. Our men of medicine can give the people the one sound reason to demand that science be allowed to release their energies today damped down because they exist half-alive.

Our physicians can give the true answer to the tories, the despisers of humanity who croak that the American people go on living in tenements and hovels because they are no good, that they lean on their shovels because they are lazy.

Medical science answers these moss-backs that they are putting the cart before the horse. Let medical science show the needed change in our human environment, and through nationwide action for human conservation bring the people the health that science now knows how to give them.

Then the American people will no longer be content to live in those miserable houses. Then twenty per cent of all the dog food now produced will no longer be sold for human consumption. Then at last the people will no longer stand it to see their pigs burned and their corn plowed under. Then they will take action on the words of their present President, who said—

"If all the nation lived on a first class diet, we would have to put more acres than we have ever cultivated into the production of an additional supply of things for Americans to eat."

For our physicians are now ready to tell the people that they cannot reach health's highest level unless they do live—all of them—on a first class diet.

This dream of our new men against death, to rebuild America on the people's demand for human conservation, will come true, sure as tomorrow's sunrise. Yet it remains a vision dimly seen, a project for the future. The immediate demands of the people are more modest ones—namely, they ask a health program to guard them from death that is needless.

Once they realize the power of today's medical science waiting to be unleashed against, for example, pneumonia, will they long remain content with any political leaders who give this or that reason for not putting a nationwide health program into action? Pneumonia is the third ranking cause of death of the American people. Right now—given the means—our doctors could make that death negligible.

Just two years ago, our political leaders could have presented an excellent alibi to the people asking to be guarded from this strangling terror. Then there was only serum to cure some of them and the cost of that serum was, for one case, about a hundred dollars.

But now have come those white pills—sulfapyridine—the cost of which is $5 for saving the life of a man or woman, and $2.50 for saving the life of a little child or a baby.

Our political leaders may be right if they protest that $100 is too much to spend for serum to save a life from pneumonia. But who dares tell the voters that $5 is too much to spend for those white pills that can save a man or woman? Or that $2.50 to save the life of a little boy or girl would put too much of a strain on the nation's pocketbook?

Here is the entering wedge that the people can use in their demand for a national health program. For only a national health program will make possible the laboratories, the public health nurses, the training of the doctors to take full advantage of this cheap new medicine's life-saving power. It is comparable to the story of the way our highway system got built, exactly. Endless propaganda and the existence of expensive limousines failed to give us good roads. The coming of the cheap flivver forced their building.

Once they understand it, the cheap and simple life-saving power of those plain white pills will put questions in the heads of the people. They will join together to ask: Why are we not all now saved from pneumonia? Who is it that distinguishes between who should live and who should die?

And it is an easy step to go from pneumonia to the same question for all sickness and death now preventable. Because for all preventable death Max Peet's simple arithmetic holds true—"It costs us less to save 'em than to bury 'em."

This justifies hope for a national program of human conservation: that men of medical science are ready to join hands with the people in their fight for life. And it is more and more the people's intent that all who can shall live. And it is the mystic aim of the stronghearts of medical science that none who can be saved shall die. To get action, we all have only this to remember: While politicians dally, death does not wait.

Index

Abell, Dr. Irvin, National Health Conference plan criticized by, 20

Accounting, public health, 207, 223-224

Alliance Review, 112

American Institute of Public Opinion poll on syphilis question, 1937, 64

American Medical Association, 58, 110, 166; Board of Trustees' examination of health plan, 110-111; committee rebuffed by Roche committee, 214; committee's conference with Surgeon General Parran, 216-219; conflict with New Deal, 111, 119-122, 185, 214-215, 224-225; indicted by Department of Justice, 111, 185, 214-215, 224-225; National Health Conference recommendations opposed by, 19-23; national health law advocated by, 117, 186-188, 213-215; progressives, 120-122; *St. Louis Star-Times'* attack on, 118-119, 121-122; Wagner health bill opposed by, 186, 233

Arteries, hardening of, 51

Arthritis, 51

Atabrine, 41

Baltimore Sun, 100

Bankers: engineer-type of, 107-108; role of, in national health program, 90-95

Blindness, syphilis as cause of, 48

Blood pressure, high, 51

Bok, Cary, 130

Breakey, Dr. Robert, 168

Brunk, Dr. A. S., 215, 218-219, 226

Bullowa, Dr. J. G. M., 27

Bundesen, Herman, 56, 226

California, group medical care in, 198

Cancer, 65, 145; clinics, 173-174; federal aid necessary in fight against, 176-177; inadequacy of facilities for treatment of, 86-87, 173, 175-176; Massachusetts' fight against, 175; New York's fight against, 160, 161; possible progress against, 72; prevalence in U. S., 46; public problem, 172-177; treatment, 55, 175

Cancer Control Act, 24

Capone, Al, 3, 5

Carstens, Dr. Henry R., 215, 218-219, 226

Charity, medical, 197-198

Charlotte (N. C.) *News*, 113

Chicago, obstetrical record of, 56

239

INDEX

Rheumatism, 145

Richmond Times Dispatch, Virginia health program urged by, 116

Rivers, Dr. Thomas M., 28

Roche, Josephine, 18-20, 96, 104, 186-187, 214

Roosevelt, Franklin D., 12; condemned at St. Louis American Medical Association convention, 120; conference with De Kruif, 225-231; *Essentials for a National Health Program* submitted to, 17-18; health of nation discussed by, 98; *Human Erosion* and *Human Conservation* submitted to, 102-104; Interdepartmental Committee instructed by, 188; medical progress praised by, 117; memorandum on health submitted to, 32-33; national diet discussed by, 235; open letter to, proposed, 36-37

Rose, Philip S., 11, 35-39, 96, 102, 226; attitude toward health program, 96-97; presides at meeting in Philadelphia, 130-132

Rumely, Dr. Edward, 114

St. Lawrence County, N. Y., maternity care in, 178-179

St. Louis Star-Times, American Medical Association attacked by, 118-119, 121-122

Sallens, Henry, interviewed, 41-42

Scarlet fever, progress against, 140-141

Schools, health inspection in, 138-139, 147

Scripps, William J., 11, 226

Sex hormones, melancholia during menopause treated by use of, 56

Silicosis, 50

Simpson, Dr. Walter M., 27

Smallpox, 147-148

Smith, Adam, 41

Social security legislation and health, 93-94, 98-99

Spastics, 145

Specialists, necessity for, 88

State health programs (*see also under various states*): budgets, 59; federal government aid in, 219-224; fundamental need in public health, 191-192, 195

Sulfanilamide, 205; gonorrhea treated with, 55

Sulfapyridine, 55, 65, 160, 166, 205, 236-237

Syphilis, 146; American Institute of Public Opinion poll on, 64; Ingham County's fight against, 167-172; New York's campaign against, 160; possible progress against, 71; prevalence in U. S., 48-49; tests in Michigan, 147, 148; treatment, 54; Wisconsin's campaign against, 75-76

Teachers, medical examination of, in Michigan, 151

Toxoid, 74

Tuberculosis, 66, 145; Detroit's campaign against, 8-14; inadequacy of facilities for treatment, 86, 203-204; na-